GROUP THERAPY FOR SUBSTANCE USE DISORDERS

Group Therapy for Substance Use Disorders

A MOTIVATIONAL COGNITIVE-BEHAVIORAL APPROACH

Linda Carter Sobell
Mark B. Sobell

THE GUILFORD PRESS
New York   London

© 2011 The Guilford Press
A Division of Guilford Publications, Inc.
72 Spring Street, New York, NY 10012
www.guilford.com

Printed in the United States of America

This book is printed on acid-free paper.

Last digit is print number: 9 8 7 6 5 4 3 2 1

The authors have checked with sources believed to be reliable in their efforts to provide information that is complete and generally in accord with the standards of practice that are accepted at the time of publication. However, in view of the possibility of human error or changes in behavioral, mental health, or medical sciences, neither the authors, nor the editor and publisher, nor any other party who has been involved in the preparation or publication of this work warrants that the information contained herein is in every respect accurate or complete, and they are not responsible for any errors or omissions or the results obtained from the use of such information. Readers are encouraged to confirm the information contained in this book with other sources.

Library of Congress Cataloging-in-Publication Data

Sobell, Linda C.
    Group therapy for substance use disorders : a motivational cognitive-behavioral approach / Linda Carter Sobell, Mark B. Sobell.
       p. ; cm.
    Includes bibliographical references and index.
    ISBN 978-1-60918-051-5 (pbk.: alk. paper)
    1. Substance abuse—Treatment.   2. Group psychotherapy.   3. Motivational interviewing.   4. Cognitive therapy.   I. Sobell, Mark B.   II. Title.
    [DNLM: 1. Substance-Related Disorders—therapy.   2. Psychotherapy, Group—methods.   WM 270 S677g 2011]
    RC564.S567 2011
    616.89′152—dc22
                                                    2010025130

This book is dedicated to four very special people in our lives.

First, to Mark's mother, Mollie, and to Linda's grandmother, Sadie,
who had a major influence on each of our lives.
We only wish they were still here so we could share this with them.

Second, to our daughters and special friends, Stacey and Kimberly,
who have enriched our lives in so many ways.

About the Authors

Linda Carter Sobell, PhD, ABPP, is Professor and Associate Director of Clinical Training at the Center for Psychological Studies at Nova Southeastern University (NSU) in Fort Lauderdale, Florida. She is also Co-Director of the Guided Self-Change Clinic at NSU. For 17 years she was a Senior Scientist at the Addiction Research Foundation (Canada) and a Professor at the University of Toronto. A Fellow of the American Psychological Association, a Motivational Interviewing Trainer, and a Diplomate in Cognitive and Behavioral Psychology of the American Board of Professional Psychology, Dr. Sobell is nationally and internationally known for her research in the addictions field, particularly brief motivational interventions, the process of self-change, and the Timeline Followback. She has given more than 300 invited presentations and workshops, published more than 275 articles and book chapters, authored seven books, serves on several editorial boards, and for over three decades has been the recipient of grants from several federal agencies. She is past president of the Association for Behavioral and Cognitive Therapies and of the Society of Clinical Psychology of the American Psychological Association. Among Dr. Sobell's awards are the Betty Ford Award from the Association for Medical Education and Research in Substance Abuse, the Norman E. Zinberg Memorial Award from Harvard University, the Distinguished Scientific Contribution Award from the Society of Clinical Psychology of the American Psychological Association, the Lifetime Achievement Award from the Addictions Special Interest Group of the Association for Behavioral and Cognitive Therapies, the Brady/Schuster Award for outstanding behavioral science research in psychopharmacology and substance abuse from Division 28 of the American Psychological Association, and the 2008 Charles C. Shepard Science Award for the most outstanding peer-reviewed research paper on prevention and control published by Centers for Disease Control and Prevention/Agency for Toxic Substances and Disease Registry scientists.

Mark B. Sobell, PhD, ABPP, is Professor and Co-Director of the Guided Self-Change Clinic at the Center for Psychological Studies at NSU. For 16 years he was a Senior Scientist at the Addiction Research Foundation (Canada) and a Professor at the University of Toronto. A Diplomate in Cognitive and Behavioral Psychology of the American Board of Professional Psychology, Dr. Sobell is nationally and internationally recognized for his work in the area of addictive behaviors, particularly brief motivational interventions, the process of self-change, and the Timeline Followback. He has given more than 200 invited presentations and workshops, published more than 275 articles and book chapters, authored six books, serves on several editorial boards, and for over three decades has been the recipient of grants from several federal agencies. He was Acting Editor of the *Journal of Consulting and Clinical Psychology* and is currently Associate Editor of *Psychology of Addictive Behaviors* and the *Journal of Consulting and Clinical Psychology*. Among Dr. Sobell's awards are the Distinguished Scientific Contribution Award from the Society of Clinical Psychology of the American Psychological Association, the 2008 Charles C. Shepard Science Award, the Lifetime Achievement Award from the Addictions Special Interest Group of the Association for Behavioral and Cognitive Therapies, and the Jellinek Memorial Award for outstanding contributions to knowledge in the field of alcohol studies.

Preface

This book emerges from a study we conducted comparing our Guided Self-Change (GSC) treatment model (M. B. Sobell & Sobell, 1993a, 2005) delivered in a group with individual therapy (L. C. Sobell, Sobell, & Agrawal, 2009). Although our initial intent was to develop, validate, and successfully extend the GSC treatment model used in individual therapy to a group setting, as discussed in Chapter 1, that extension presented some unexpected challenges.

Our objectives in writing this book were (1) to describe how to effectively conduct and manage the dynamics of interpersonal interactions in groups (e.g., structure of groups, developing cohesion, handling difficult clients) with clients with substance use disorders; (2) to demonstrate how to integrate the basic principles of cognitive-behavioral therapy and motivational interviewing into group therapy; (3) to discuss how to manage difficult and challenging clinical situations and issues that arise when conducting groups; and (4) to present a brief overview of the treatment outcome results of our randomized clinical trial comparing the GSC treatment model in group and individual formats. In the latter regard, this book provided an opportunity to update the GSC treatment that was presented in our earlier book (M. B. Sobell & Sobell, 1993a).

The terms *patient* and *client* are used interchangeably throughout this book, as both terms are used in clinical psychology and behavioral health. When presenting clinical examples, we have removed all identifying information, and for consistency we refer to male clients as *Bill* and to female clients as *Mary*.

INTEGRATION OF CLINICAL MATERIAL AND DIALOGUE INTO THE TEXT

Almost all of the clinical materials and questionnaires, as well as therapist and client handouts, are integrated into the chapters rather than included as appendices. This makes the clinical material more user friendly, clinically useful, and easier to access. Chapter 3 describes the assessment with a discussion of the clinical utility of the measures and instruments used, including sample therapist dialogues illustrating how to discuss the assessment with clients. Chapter

4 discusses the GSC treatment delivered in an individual format and provides session outlines for therapists that include objectives, procedures, and materials and handouts needed. Chapter 5 similarly presents session outlines for therapists for each group session. In addition, Chapter 5 includes sample round-robin discussions. Clinical examples are included throughout the book, and particularly in Part II, that demonstrate (1) how to implement the GSC treatment model in both individual and group therapy and (2) how to integrate cognitive-behavioral and motivational interviewing strategies and techniques into group therapy, including the assessment measures and questionnaires and associated motivational interviewing feedback materials.

INTENDED AUDIENCE

This book has two intended audiences. The first is practitioners and clinicians who are already treating individuals with substance use problems and who want to learn how to successfully integrate cognitive-behavioral and motivational interviewing techniques into group therapy. The second audience is practitioners and clinicians not in the substance abuse field who want to learn more about how to conduct and manage the dynamics of interpersonal interactions in groups and how to integrate cognitive-behavioral and motivational interviewing principles and techniques into group therapy. We hope that those reading this book will come away with an appreciation that, although group therapy is more complex and challenging than individual therapy, it is also extremely rewarding and can accomplish things not easily achieved in individual treatment.

Acknowledgments

This book is based on a randomized clinical trial that evaluated the Guided Self-Change (GSC) treatment model in a group- versus an individual-therapy format. It was conducted when we directed the GSC Unit at the Addiction Research Foundation in Toronto, Canada. We wish to thank Dr. Joan Marshman, who at the time was the Foundation President, and the GSC staff, who contributed to the success of the study (in alphabetical order): Sangeeta Agrawal, Margaret Beardwood, Diane Benedek, Curtis Breslin, Joanne Brown, Barbara Bruce, Giao Buchan, Carole Bush, Virginia Chow, Pat Cleland, John Cunningham, Judy Dobson, Doug Gavin, Joanne Jackson, Lisa Johnson-Young, Mel Kahan, Even Kwan, Gloria Leo, Eric Rubel, Lorna Sagorsky, Kathy Sdao-Jarvie, Peter Selby, Jennifer-Ann Shillingford, Joanne Spratt, Kathy Voros, Peter Voros, Lynn Wilson, and Kim Zynck. In addition, we want to thank all our doctoral students at the Center for Psychological Studies at Nova Southeastern University in Fort Lauderdale, Florida, who, as part of their training, were supervised by us in the conduct of group therapy. Because of that supervision over the past 12 years, we have continued to refine our approach to conducting group therapy and to applying motivational interviewing techniques in a group setting.

Several years ago, we attended two workshops presented by Dr. Robert Dies that greatly influenced our approach to group therapy. As will be evident after reading this book, what influenced us most were the concepts of *Think Group*, the *Music Comes from the Group*, and *Therapists as Conductors*. Furthermore, his suggestions for handling difficult and challenging clients and group situations have proven invaluable. A special thanks to Anaeli Ramos, Jessica Ruiz, Rachael Silverman, and Andrew Voluse for their help with the preparation of the book manuscript. Thanks to Sir Meowy for keeping us company and sitting on the manuscript pages late at night. In addition, we want to thank the many clients who over the years participated in our groups, as they taught us a great deal about groups and group processes. Dr. Beverly Thorn's book *Cognitive Therapy for Chronic Pain* (2004) also provided some very useful ideas about how to present the clinical materials in this book.

We also are indebted to William R. Miller, a consummate scientist/clinician, who masterfully formalized the major elements of motivational interviewing. Motivational interviewing has been an increasingly important component of our approach and is an important pillar of the treatment approach in this book.

Last, we are indebted to Jim Nageotte, our editor at The Guilford Press, for his patience and support. Although, from our perspective, the final product was never in doubt, it took far longer to complete than we anticipated. In this regard, we want to thank Jim for not abandoning this project. Finally, a special thanks to an anonymous reviewer of the book manuscript whose detailed comments led to a more reader-friendly and clinically useful book.

Contents

APPENDICES

List of Figures, Tables, and Therapist and Client Handouts

FIGURES

TABLES

THERAPIST HANDOUTS

CLIENT HANDOUTS

PART I

Rationale, Research, and Assessment

CHAPTER 1

Guided Self-Change Treatment and Its Successful Extension to Group Therapy

> A persuasive body of outcome research has demonstrated unequivocally that group therapy is a highly effectively form of psychotherapy and that it is at least equal to individual psychotherapy in its power to provide meaningful benefit.
> —YALOM AND LESZCZ (2005, p. 1)

This chapter lays the foundation for the rest of this book by (1) reviewing the development of the Guided Self-Change (GSC) treatment model and the several lines of research that influenced the model; (2) comparing the GSC treatment model with other cognitive-behavioral interventions for substance use disorders; (3) discussing how the GSC treatment model was successfully disseminated throughout the community in which it was originally developed; and (4) presenting the results of the randomized controlled trial (RCT) that successfully extended the GSC treatment model developed as an individual treatment to a group therapy format.

The GSC treatment model was an outgrowth of our earlier research on outpatient treatment of problem drinkers. In comparison with more severely dependent drinkers, problem drinkers are not physiologically dependent on alcohol, tend to have had a problem for fewer years, are usually employed, have a supportive environment, and are very resistant to traditional labels such as *alcoholic* or *drug addict*. These differences are described in detail in our earlier book, *Problem Drinkers: Guided Self-Change Treatment* (M. B. Sobell & Sobell, 1993a). Although the GSC treatment model was developed for English-speaking problem drinkers, it has been extended to and evaluated with drug abusers whose problems are not severe (L. C. Sobell et al., 2009; L. C. Sobell, Wagner, Sobell, Agrawal, & Ellingstad, 2006) and to Spanish-speaking alcohol abusers (Ayala, Echeverría, Sobell, & Sobell, 1997, 1998; Ayala-Velazquez, Cardenas, Echeverría, & Gutierrez, 1995). The findings of our study comparing GSC delivered in a group versus an individual-treatment format and extending the GSC treatment model to drug abusers are presented in this chapter, as is a summary of a previous review of several studies that evaluated the GSC treatment model and adaptations of that model (M. B. Sobell & Sobell, 2005).

INFLUENCES ON THE DEVELOPMENT OF THE GSC TREATMENT MODEL

As reviewed elsewhere (M. B. Sobell & Sobell, 1993a, 2005), several lines of research influenced the development of the GSC treatment model. The first major influence derived from epidemiological research conducted in the 1970s showing that many individuals had alcohol problems that were not severe (e.g., Cahalan & Room, 1974; Schuckit, Smith, Danko, Bucholz, & Reich, 2001; M. B. Sobell & Sobell, 1993b). Consistent with other health problems, it seemed reasonable to think such individuals might benefit from a less intense, briefer intervention compared with individuals with more severe alcohol problems. Related to this was research on problem drinkers' preferences for moderation goals (Heather & Robertson, 1981; Marlatt et al., 1985; Miller, 1986–1987).

Another important influence on the development of the GSC treatment model was a study by Edwards and his colleagues (1977) that found that one session of advice or counseling produced the same outcomes as a comprehensive treatment. Furthermore, individuals randomly assigned to either condition generally showed considerable improvement. Although the majority of cognitive-behavioral studies until that time had emphasized skills training, improvement following a single session could not be explained by skills training. Rather, the most likely explanation was that many individuals have the capacity to change their substance abuse problem if sufficiently motivated and that the single session catalyzed their motivation. Such thinking is supported by research on the phenomenon of self-change (i.e., natural recovery) that has shown that many people with alcohol and drug problems can successfully change on their own (reviewed in Klingemann & Sobell, 2007).

Bandura's (1977, 1986) social cognitive theory was another influence on the development of the GSC treatment model, as it suggested that self-efficacy, outcome expectations, and goal choice might be important determinants of motivation. Many individuals with substance use disorders (SUDs), especially those whose problems are not severe, are ambivalent about the need to change. In this regard, another influence was the development of motivational interviewing, a therapeutic approach put forth by Miller and his colleagues to minimize resistance and increase clients' motivation to change (Miller, 1983; Miller & Rollnick, 1991, 2002). The motivational interviewing approach was consistent with Prochaska and DiClemente's (1984) transtheoretical model of change that conceptualized motivation as a state and targeted increasing motivation for change as a focus of therapy. For these reasons, motivational interviewing has become the recommended counseling style for developing a therapeutic alliance with clients (Kazdin, 2007; Meier, Barrowclough, & Donmall, 2005; Moyers, Miller, & Hendrickson, 2005).

THE GSC TREATMENT MODEL COMPARED WITH OTHER COGNITIVE-BEHAVIORAL INTERVENTIONS FOR SUDs

The GSC intervention reflects a synergy of time-tested cognitive-behavioral strategies that are delivered using motivational interviewing techniques (e.g., rolling with resistance, decisional balance exercise, readiness ruler). Although the GSC treatment model has several unique features, it also shares many features with other cognitive-behavioral interventions, including the use of functional analysis (M. B. Sobell, Sobell, & Sheahan, 1976); self-monitoring of alcohol and drug use (L. C. Sobell & Sobell, 1973); problem-solving skills to develop alternative responses to drinking or drug use situations (D'Zurilla & Goldfried, 1971); and homework assignments, including a decisional balance exercise (Janis & Mann, 1977; Kazantzis, Deane, & Ronan, 2000).

Table 1.1 highlights the major differences between the GSC treatment model and other cognitive-behavioral interventions for SUDs. Factors unique to the GSC treatment model include (1) incorporating cognitive elements of the relapse prevention model (Marlatt & Donovan, 2005; Marlatt & Gordon, 1985; M. B. Sobell & Sobell, 1993a); (2) allowing alcohol clients to self-select their treatment goals (i.e., moderation or abstinence; M. B. Sobell & Sobell, 1995); (3) using the Timeline Followback (TLFB) to provide clients with feedback about their pretreatment alcohol or drug use and related risks (Agrawal, Sobell, & Sobell, 2008; L. C. Sobell & Sobell, 2003); (4) allowing clients to request additional sessions after the four semistructured GSC sessions (M. B. Sobell & Sobell, 1993a); and (5) using a motivational interviewing style throughout the delivery of the intervention.

Before we further describe the GSC treatment model and its extension to group therapy, it is important to briefly review the findings of studies that compared the same treatment delivered in individual and group formats with substance abusers. As will be apparent, such studies are few in number.

BRIEF REVIEW OF STUDIES COMPARING GROUP AND INDIVIDUAL TREATMENTS FOR SUDs

With a long and rich history (Bernard & MacKenzie, 1994; Scheidlinger, 1994; Yalom & Leszcz, 2005), group therapy is a popular form of treatment across many clinical disciplines (e.g., psychology, psychiatry, social work) and across a wide range of clinical problems (e.g., anxiety and mood disorders, posttraumatic stress disorder, obesity) (Barlow, Burlingame, Nebeker, & Ander-

---

TABLE 1.1. Major Ways the GSC Treatment Model Differs from Other Cognitive-Behavioral Interventions for SUDs

- Provides goal choice that includes low-risk drinking and accepts harm-reduction alternatives for clients not willing to seek abstinence.

- Clients functionally analyze their own substance use (i.e., identify high-risk trigger situations and associated consequences for use) and develop their own treatment plans.

- Emphasizes the application of problem-solving skills.

- Incorporates cognitive elements of the relapse prevention model into the treatment. Rather than providing skills training, a relapse management approach is used to generate a dialogue about taking a realistic perspective on change and to discuss the need to construe slips as learning experiences.

- Uses the Timeline Followback to gather pretreatment substance use data that are then used to generate personalized feedback for clients about their level of substance use, risks, and consequences.

- Incorporates flexibility in scheduling, explicitly soliciting client input as the main determinant for additional sessions.

- As a brief intervention, it includes an aftercare telephone call 1 month after the last scheduled session that is intended to provide support for clients' functioning and to facilitate resumption of treatment if needed.

- Uses motivational interviewing as a communication style throughout the intervention, in addition to incorporating various motivational interviewing strategies and techniques (e.g., readiness ruler, advice feedback, decisional balancing).

son, 2000; Guimon, 2004; Humphreys et al., 2004; Panas, Caspi, Fournier, & McCarty, 2003; Satterfield, 1994; Scheidlinger, 1994; Weiss, Jaffee, deMenil, & Cogley, 2004). In the substance abuse field it is the "most common treatment modality" (Weiss et al., 2004, p. 339). The popularity of groups relates in large part to two factors: (1) the provision of social support to clients and (2) the ability to treat multiple clients concurrently and at a lower cost than individual therapy.

The term *group therapy* has been used to describe a wide variety of therapeutic activities (e.g., educational, didactic, interactional, process, support, aftercare, codependency), including self-help groups. Although self-help groups, a widely used group format in the substance abuse field, incorporate and resemble some aspects of group therapy, there are several major differences, the most significant being that leaders need no professional training (Scheidlinger, 1994; Yalom & Leszcz, 2005). Consequently, self-help groups are not included in this review.

Group therapy has a long tradition in the treatment of SUDs (Center for Substance Abuse Treatment, 2005; Institute of Medicine, 1990; Panas et al., 2003; Vannicelli, 1992; Weiss et al., 2004), especially with adolescents (D'Amico et al., 2011; Kaminer, 2005). Given this history, one might expect to find considerable research supporting the efficacy of group therapy with SUDs. To the contrary, RCTs of group versus individual treatment are sparse and lack appropriate controls (Institute of Medicine, 1990; Weiss et al., 2004).

In one of the first reviews of the group therapy literature with alcohol abusers, Brandsma and Pattison (1985) found 30 studies. Based on their review, they concluded that it was impossible to evaluate the efficacy of group therapy, as the research was plagued with multiple problems (e.g., inadequate designs, inadequate specification of procedures, lack of controls, poor measures, lack of replications), including that most of the group treatments had been combined with other program components (e.g., individual therapy, aftercare, self-help meetings). Despite these problems, the studies reported abstinence or improvement rates ranging from 15 to 53%, comparable to those for individual treatments.

A similar review conducted two decades later (Weiss et al., 2004) found that little has changed from the Brandsma and Pattison (1985) review. In this recent review, 24 comparative trials of group therapy with SUDs were found. The authors classified these studies into six distinct categories: (1) group therapy versus no group therapy (e.g., Stephens, Roffman, & Curtin, 2000); (2) group therapy versus individual therapy (e.g., Marques & Formigoni, 2001); (3) group therapy plus individual therapy versus group therapy alone (e.g., Linehan et al., 1999); (4) group therapy plus individual therapy versus individual therapy alone (e.g., McKay et al., 1997); (5) group therapy versus another group therapy with different content or theoretical orientation (e.g., Kadden, Cooney, Getter, & Litt, 1989); and (6) more group therapy versus less group therapy (e.g., Coviello et al., 2001). The two major conclusions from this review were that no significant outcome differences existed between group and individual treatments and that no single type of group therapy was superior.

RCTs of the Same Treatment Delivered in a Group versus Individual Format for SUDs

Because the RCT of the GSC treatment model involved an evaluation of the same treatment in an individual versus a group format (L. C. Sobell et al., 2009), the following review includes only RCTs that compare the same treatment delivered in a group versus an individual format. Consequently, studies comparing different types of groups (e.g., Abrams & Wilson, 1979; Miller & Taylor, 1980; Oei & Jackson, 1980) or different group and individual treatments (e.g., McKay et al., 1997; Stephens et al., 2000) are not included. In addition, family and marital studies are excluded, as they have no individual-treatment component.

Of the 24 studies in the Weiss and colleagues (2004) review, only 3 (12.5%) addressed the efficacy of group compared with individual therapy for SUDs (Graham, Annis, Brett, & Venesoen, 1996; Marques & Formigoni, 2001; Schmitz et al., 1997). Although not in the Weiss and colleagues review, a fourth study (Duckert, Johnsen, & Amundsen, 1992) using an RCT compared the same treatment in group and individual formats for alcohol abusers. To facilitate comparisons among these four RCTs, the major characteristics of each study are listed in Table 1.2. Thus only details not in Table 1.2 are discussed subsequently.

In the Graham and colleagues (1996) study, alcohol and drug abusers were randomized to 12 sessions of relapse prevention aftercare treatment delivered in either a group or an individual format. At the follow-up, there were no significant differences between the two treatment conditions on any alcohol or drug use outcome measures. However, prior to randomization, all clients had participated in one of two treatment programs for SUDs (12-step 26-day residential program or 1-year outpatient eclectic group). Because other interventions (mainly groups) immediately preceded this study's comparison of group and individual aftercare, it does not allow a true comparison of the efficacy of the two aftercare treatment modalities.

TABLE 1.2. RCTs of the Same Treatment Delivered in Group versus Individual Formats for SUDs

	Author (year)			
Study characteristic	Duckert et al. (1992)	Graham et al. (1996)	Marques & Formigoni (2001)	Schmitz et al. (1997)
Country	Norway	Canada	Brazil	United States
Sample size	135	192	155	32
% Male	60.0	66.9	92.0	50.0
Type of substance abuse problem	Alcohol	Alcohol and other drugs	Alcohol and other drugs	Cocaine
Treatment type	Cognitive-behavioral	Relapse prevention aftercare	Cognitive-behavioral	Cognitive-behavioral relapse prevention aftercare
No. of scheduled sessions	12	12	17	12
Length (min) of group sessions	90	60–90	—	60
Follow-up period (mo)	21	12	15	6
% Found for follow-up	57.7	74.0	68.4	84.0
Self-reports confirmed	Yes	No	Yes	Yes
Significant outcome differences				
Pre- versus posttreatment	Yes	Yes	Yes	Yes
Group versus individual	No	No	No	No

Note. Dash indicates that data were not reported.

In the Schmitz and colleagues (1997) study, cocaine-dependent clients who had recently completed an inpatient chemical dependency treatment program were subsequently randomly assigned (by cohorts) to a 12-session manualized cognitive-behavioral relapse prevention treatment delivered in either a group or individual format. At the follow-up, there were no significant differences between the two conditions. As with the Graham and colleagues (1996) study, because all participants had received other substance abuse treatment before the RCT, a pure test of the efficacy of the two aftercare treatments is not possible.

In the Marques and Formigoni (2001) study, alcohol and drug abusers were randomly assigned to a 17-session cognitive-behavioral treatment delivered in either a group or an individual format. The first treatment session, which was conducted individually for both conditions, consisted of reviewing assessment data and presenting educational information about alcohol and drugs. Abstinence was required of all participants for the first 3 months, after which alcohol clients could select a moderation goal. Although the two conditions did not have significantly different outcomes at the follow-up, 7% of participants had dropped out after the first session, and only 54% completed 8 of the 17 sessions. Although there were no significant differences in dropout rates between the group and individual conditions, drug clients attended significantly fewer sessions than did alcohol clients.

In the Duckert and colleagues (1992) study, alcohol abusers were recruited through newspaper advertisements, matched pairwise, and then randomly assigned to a 12-session cognitive-behavioral treatment delivered in either a group or an individual format. Groups were of a single gender, and all participants were allowed to select an abstinence or moderation drinking goal. Besides the format, the two conditions differed in the number of hours spent in sessions (individual: 7 hours; group: 25 hours). At follow-up no significant differences were found between the group and individual conditions on a number of outcome variables, including alcohol consumption. When asked at the follow-up, a larger number of group than individual participants reported that they wanted more contact with their therapists. This may reflect the feeling that group participants had received proportionately less personal attention from their therapists than they would have if they had been assigned to individual therapy.

In summary, RCTs comparing the same treatment delivered in a group versus an individual format for clients with SUDs are rare. Of the four published studies, two (Graham et al., 1996; Schmitz et al., 1997) were not pure comparisons, as clients had received other treatment immediately prior to being randomized. The most striking and consistent finding across all four studies, however, was that, although clients demonstrated significant improvements in their substance use, there were no differences between the group- and individual-treatment formats. Last, none of the four studies reported any cost-effectiveness evaluations of group versus individual treatment.

Research Issues in Conducting RCTs of Group versus Individual Therapy

Several issues make it difficult to conduct research studies comparing group with individual therapy. One serious problem that can threaten the validity of such treatment comparisons is differential attrition (Piper, 1993; Piper & Joyce, 1996). In this regard, studies have shown that a greater number of clients drop out when assigned to group than to individual therapy (Budman et al., 1988; Hofmann & Suvak, 2006). The Budman and colleagues (1988) study, an RCT of group versus individual therapy with psychiatric clients, illustrates the importance of implementing strategies to minimize dropouts. The great majority of the 29 patients who dropped out after being informed of their assignment had been assigned to group rather than individual therapy (89.7%, $n = 26$; 10.3%, $n = 3$, respectively). Therefore, although significant improvements occurred in both conditions, it was impossible to draw firm conclusions about the relative efficacy of group versus individual therapy because of differential attrition. Another issue concerns recruiting a sufficient number of participants to randomize to group and individual treatment, particularly in closed groups (i.e., those to which no new members are added after the first session), which can be difficult. Other complicating factors involve group characteristics (e.g., gender composition) and different session lengths for group and individual therapy. Last, a critical issue that must be addressed in any comparative evaluation of group versus individual treatment is whether the study is a pure comparison in which there are no other concurrent or preceding treatment components (e.g., treatments preceding aftercare, self-help groups, pharmacotherapy) that could provide alternative explanations for the findings.

Several conclusions about the role and utility of group therapy can be drawn based on this chapter: (1) group processes play an important role in the efficacy of groups; (2) because of their inherent structure, groups offer important advantages that do not exist in an individual therapy setting; (3) groups that incorporate group processes have reported comparable outcomes to individual therapy; and (4) groups can treat multiple patients at one time, thereby reducing the financial burden on the payer. Given the widespread use of group therapy in clinical practice with SUDs, the only curious issue is why there is a paucity of research (particularly RCTs) evaluating the *same type of treatment* (e.g., theoretical orientation, procedures, number of sessions) delivered in a group versus an individual setting. With these caveats in mind, we now return to a consideration of GSC and how it was adapted to a group format.

GENERAL FRAMEWORK OF THE GSC TREATMENT MODEL

The general framework for the GSC treatment model is an assessment and four semistructured sessions, with additional sessions available as needed. The major components of a GSC assessment and four-session treatment program for substance abusers, whether delivered in an individual or a group format, are described in detail in Chapters 4 and 5, respectively. These chapters include therapist handouts for each individual therapy (4.1–4.4) and each group therapy (5.1–5.4) session. Each handout contains detailed session guidelines, objectives, procedures, and homework exercises. In addition, each group therapist handout contains guidelines on how to conduct several round-robin discussions, which is the format used to conduct the clinical intervention in a group format. Round-robin discussions were designed so that support, feedback, and advice emanate primarily from group members rather than from the group leaders.

EXTENDING THE GSC TREATMENT MODEL TO A GROUP FORMAT

The primary empirical support for the cognitive-behavioral, motivational interviewing group therapy approach that is the subject of this book derives from an RCT that compared a GSC intervention delivered in a group versus an individual format (L. C. Sobell et al., 2009). For two decades starting in the mid-1970s, our clinical research focused on developing and validating individual therapies for those with SUDs. However, by the early 1990s the substance abuse field as well as the agency where we were then employed, the Addiction Research Foundation in Toronto, Canada, had developed waiting lists for clients requesting individual therapy. At this same time, both in the United States and in Canada, there were serious concerns about health care cost containment as well as cost-effective treatments (Rosenberg & Zimet, 1995; Spitz, 2001; Steenberger & Budman, 1996). Consequently, we decided to extend and validate the GSC treatment model in a group format. The group-versus-individual study, also known as *GRIN* (*GR*oup vs. *IN*dividual), was an RCT that evaluated the GSC treatment model delivered in a group versus an individual format with 264 alcohol and drug abusers voluntarily seeking treatment. This was also the first study to evaluate the GSC treatment model with drug abusers whose problems were not severe (e.g., no intravenous drug users participated). Although discussion of the group treatment procedures and details occupies much of this book, it will be helpful to first discuss how the GRIN study evolved and to present the results of the RCT of GSC used in group and individual therapy.

All of the therapists who participated in the GRIN study were trained in conducting GSC treatment, a time-limited cognitive-behavioral motivational intervention (M. B. Sobell & Sobell, 1993a, 2005), with individual clients, and most had some, albeit limited, experience in conducting groups. However, early during a pilot study intended to precede the formal study, it became clear that the integration of cognitive-behavioral procedures (e.g., homework, self-monitoring, functional analyses of behaviors, relapse prevention) and motivational interviewing techniques, vital elements of the GSC individual treatment model, would require careful thought and attention if they were to be successfully incorporated into a group setting. The major concern was addressing the needs and problems of multiple clients while capitalizing on group processes without a loss of therapeutic effectiveness. To address this concern, we stopped the pilot study and spent several months reviewing the group psychotherapy literature to determine how to best integrate the GSC intervention into a group format. Our goal was to retain the curative elements of the GSC intervention delivered individually while addressing the constraints and opportunities intrinsic to group therapy.

After stopping the initial pilot study and providing the GSC staff with training in group skills and how to integrate them with their cognitive-behavioral and motivational interviewing skills, a second pilot study was conducted, followed by the completion of the GRIN study. We believe that the success of the GRIN study, and especially the high level of group cohesion achieved, demonstrates that we were able to successfully integrate cognitive-behavioral and motivational interviewing principles and techniques with group processes.

HOW WELL DOES GSC WORK?

As reviewed elsewhere (M. B. Sobell & Sobell, 2005), the GSC treatment model has been evaluated in multiple settings (e.g., outpatient alcohol treatment programs, primary care centers), with different populations (adults, adolescents, alcohol and drug abusers, gamblers), and with both English and Spanish speakers. A summary of the main findings of studies evaluating the GSC treatment model for clients with alcohol problems that also had 1 year or more of follow-up appears in Table 1.3. This table lists the outcome variables assessed in each study and shows the percentage change for those variables from pretreatment to posttreatment. For proportion of days abstinent, a positive change indicates improvement, whereas for mean drinks per drinking day (or mean drinks per week), a negative change indicates improvement. The amount of change demonstrated in these studies is similar to that shown in other studies of brief interventions (Babor et al., 2006) and primary care interventions (Fleming, Barry, Manwell, Johnson, & London, 1997).

There are two additional published studies, involving adolescents, that used the GSC treatment model, but because they did not meet the 1-year follow-up criterion, they are not listed in Table 1.3. In one study (Breslin, Li, Sdao-Jarvie, Tupker, & Ittig-Deland, 2002), at the 6-month follow-up, 50 adolescent substance users treated with an adaptation of GSC were found to have reduced their substance use by about 44%. The second study, also an adaptation of GSC, involved 213 African American and Hispanic adolescents. Preliminary follow-up results around 11 weeks found that clients' self-reported marijuana and alcohol use had decreased about 55% and 47%, respectively (Gil, Wagner, & Tubman, 2004). The findings from these two studies are consistent with those in Table 1.3 that have a 1-year follow-up, but they showed greater change scores, possibly because of their shorter follow-up intervals. Although studies using motivational interviewing in groups with adolescents are few in number, D'Amico and her colleagues have offered compelling arguments (D'Amico et al., 2011) and support (D'Amico, Osilla, & Hunter, in press) for motivational interviewing is particularly suited (e.g., taking a collaborative approach, addressing ambivalence about changing, avoiding labels, allowing youths to give voice to the need to change rather than being told what to do) for at-risk youths and particularly those from disadvantaged/marginalized or cultural minority backgrounds.

Because this book is intended as a clinical guide, the studies in Table 1.3 are not further discussed. The evidence, however, shows that the GSC treatment model has consistently been associated with substantial and significant gains over the course of treatment and that these changes are maintained following treatment.

How Well Does GSC Work in Groups?

Findings from the GRIN study are briefly summarized here, as they have been reported in detail elsewhere (L. C. Sobell et al., 2009). The participants had voluntarily sought treatment for an alcohol or drug problem at the Addiction Research Foundation in Toronto, Ontario, Canada. When the study was conducted, the Addiction Research Foundation was the largest outpatient service provider in the province of Ontario. The GRIN study was designed for problem drinkers and for drug abusers voluntarily seeking treatment (drug abusers who used drugs intravenously or who used heroin were excluded). The major procedural details of the GRIN study (i.e., session dialogues, forms, exercises, round-robin discussions) are described in other places throughout this book. Chapter 3 discusses assessment measures and materials used in both the GSC individual and group sessions and Chapters 4 and 5 present the GSC treatment model in terms of its application to the conduct of the individual and group therapy, respectively. Also included in these chapters are the therapist and client handouts, clinical examples, and sample therapist and client dialogues. The details of the statistical analyses of the GRIN are reported elsewhere (L. C. Sobell et al., 2009). What follows is a summary of the important findings and also some insights into the study that go beyond what can be communicated in journal articles.

The most important result of the GRIN study was that participants in both the individual- and group-treatment conditions showed sizeable and significant improvement across treatment and follow-up. There were, however, no significant differences between the two treatment formats. That is, although clients in both treatment conditions significantly reduced their alcohol or drug use, it did not matter whether they were in individual or group therapy.

TABLE 1.3. Summary of Outcome Studies Evaluating the GSC Treatment Model for Clients with Alcohol Problems

Study and group	Variable	Pretreatment	Posttreatment	Change
Andréasson, Hansagi, & Oesterlund (2002)				
4GSCS ($n = 30$)	Mean drinks/DD	5.2	4.5	−13%
1GSCS ($n = 29$)	Mean drinks/DD	6.3	4.7	−25%
Ayala et al. (1998)				
INDIV ($n = 177$)	Prop abstinent	0.73	0.82	+9%
INDIV ($n = 177$)	Mean drinks/DD	9.2	6.5	−29%
Breslin et al. (1998)				
SC ($n = 33$)	Prop abstinent	0.28	0.45	+17%
NSC ($n = 36$)	Prop abstinent	0.24	0.37	+13%
M. B. Sobell, Sobell, & Gavin (1995)				
BC ($n = 36$)	Prop abstinent	0.32	0.61	+29%
RP ($n = 33$)	Prop abstinent	0.33	0.50	+17%
BC ($n = 36$)	Mean drinks/DD	6.7	4.2	−37%
RP ($n = 33$)	Mean drinks/DD	5.1	3.6	−29%
M. B. Sobell, Sobell, & Leo (2000)				
DSS ($n = 19$)	Prop abstinent	0.23	0.47	+24%
NSS ($n = 24$)	Prop abstinent	0.21	0.44	+23%
DSS ($n = 19$)	Mean drinks/DD	6.3	4.3	−21%
NSS ($n = 24$)	Mean drinks/DD	5.8	4.6	−20%
L. C. Sobell et al. (2009)				
INDIV ($n = 107$)	Prop abstinent	0.30	0.58	+28%
GRP ($n = 105$)	Prop abstinent	0.30	0.53	+23%
INDIV ($n = 107$)	Mean drinks/DD	6.4	4.1	−36%
GRP ($n = 105$)	Mean drinks/DD	6.7	4.6	−31%
L. C. Sobell et al. (2002)				
ME/PF ($n = 321$)	Prop abstinent	0.21	0.35	+14%
B/DG ($n = 336$)	Prop abstinent	0.23	0.34	+11%
ME/PF ($n = 321$)	Mean drinks/DD	5.9	4.7	+20%
B/DG ($n = 336$)	Mean drinks/DD	5.9	4.7	+20%

Note. All studies had to have a minimum of 1 year of follow-up. Study and group designations: 4GSCS, 4 GSC sessions; 1GSCS, 1 GSC session; INDIV, individual treatment; SC, supplemental care; NSC, no supplemental care; BC, behavioral counseling; RP, behavioral counseling plus cognitive relapse prevention; DSS, directed social support; NSS, natural social support; GRP, group treatment; ME/PF, motivational enhancement/personalized feedback; B/DG, bibliotherapy/drinking guidelines. Prop abstinent, proportion of days abstinent; Mean drinks/DD, mean number of drinks consumed per drinking day. Change is defined as the percentage of change pretreatment to posttreatment. From M. B. Sobell and L. C. Sobell (2005, p. 205). Copyright 2005 by the Springer Publishing Company. Reprinted by permission.

Validity of Self-Reports and Treatment Integrity Checks

As part of the study, each participant provided the name of a collateral informant who could be contacted to corroborate the participant's self-reports of posttreatment alcohol or drug use. Results showed that collaterals confirmed participants' self-reports of alcohol and drug use (L. C. Sobell et al., 2009). A treatment integrity check on therapists' compliance with the study protocol found that compliance was uniformly high for both the individual and group treatment conditions (L. C. Sobell et al., 2009).

Outcomes for Alcohol Clients

Figure 1.1 shows that for clients who had a primary alcohol problem, the percentage of abstinent days for those in the individual and group treatment conditions were similar at all three time points. Furthermore, for clients in both conditions, the percentage of abstinent days showed a large increase over treatment that was sustained over the 12-month follow-up. Figure 1.2 shows similar results but for mean number of standard drinks consumed per drinking day. Again, the data for clients in both treatment conditions were very similar. Because some reports in the alcohol literature have noted that females have shown better outcomes than males in brief cognitive-behavioral interventions (Sanchez-Craig, Leigh, Spivak, & Lei, 1989; Sanchez-Craig, Spivak, & Davila, 1991), we explored whether there were any gender differences. However, no significant differences related to gender or relating gender to treatment conditions were found for this study.

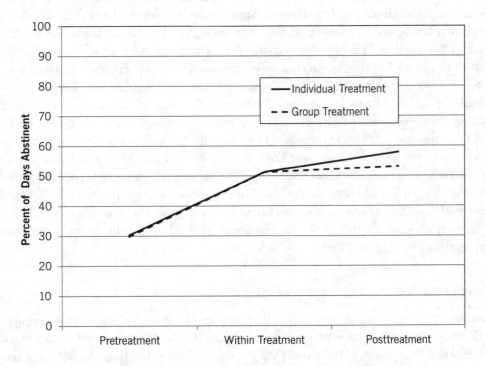

FIGURE 1.1. Percent of days abstinent during pretreatment, within treatment, and posttreatment for problem drinkers assigned to individual- and group-treatment conditions.

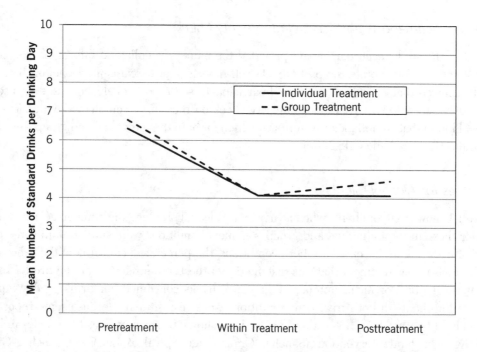

FIGURE 1.2. Mean number of standard drinks per drinking day during pretreatment, within treatment, and posttreatment for problem drinkers assigned to individual- and group-treatment conditions.

For clients with alcohol problems, an interesting pattern of improvement was observed. As in other studies involving problem drinkers, approximately three-quarters of the clients chose to work on reducing rather than stopping their drinking (Sanchez-Craig, Annis, Bornet, & Mac-Donald, 1984; M. B. Sobell, Sobell, & Gavin, 1995). However, in terms of drinking outcomes, as shown in Figure 1.3, the main change over the course of treatment and follow-up was that alcohol clients greatly reduced their percentage of heavy drinking days (i.e., five or more standard drinks), and concurrently increased their percentage of abstinent days. In contrast, their frequency of limited drinking days (i.e., one to four standard drinks) stayed almost constant from pre- to posttreatment. This phenomenon, in which clients chose a low-risk, limited-drinking goal but then increased their abstinent days, is consistent with another study (Sanchez-Craig, 1980) that found that those assigned to a low-risk drinking goal were significantly better able to abstain for the first 3 weeks of treatment (they were requested to do so putatively to facilitate the assessment) than those randomly assigned to an abstinence goal. These findings strongly suggest that the way clients view their ability to manage their drinking can be an important variable affecting their drinking decisions.

Outcomes for Cocaine and Cannabis Clients

In addition to providing a demonstration that the GSC intervention delivered in groups was as effective as the same intervention delivered individually, the GRIN study also extended the GSC treatment model to individuals with drug problems other than alcohol, most notably cocaine and cannabis. Figure 1.4 shows how the percentage of days abstinent from drug use changed from pretreatment through treatment and follow-up. Because there were no significant

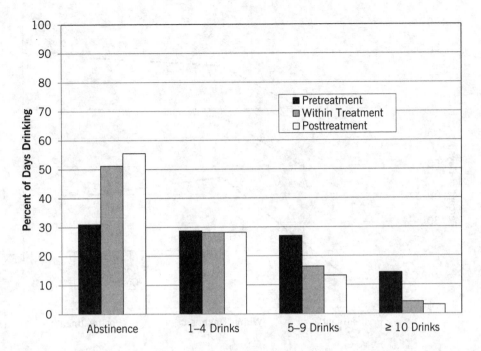

FIGURE 1.3. Percent of days drinking at different levels during pretreatment, within treatment, and posttreatment for problem drinkers. Because the individual- and group-treatment conditions did not differ significantly, they were combined.

differences at any point between clients in the group or individual conditions, data from both conditions were combined in Figure 1.4. As can be seen, clients with a primary cocaine problem improved considerably over treatment and continued to improve over follow-up. For clients for whom cannabis was the primary problem, although substantial gains over treatment were made, some regression over the follow-up year occurred. At the end of follow-up, however, they still were using far less than prior to treatment.

Therapist Time Ratio Analysis of GSC Group versus Individual Treatment

When treatments that require different amounts of resources are compared, the key question is not whether one treatment is as effective as another but whether a more expensive or demanding treatment (from the patient's perspective) produces sufficiently superior outcomes to warrant the added cost or personal investment. In evaluating the GSC treatment in a group versus an individual format, we calculated a therapist time ratio comparing the time spent providing group compared with individual treatment. This evaluation showed that there was a 41.4% savings in therapists' time when conducting group therapy (L. C. Sobell et al., 2009).

Clients' Evaluations of the GSC Intervention at the End of Treatment

Almost all of the participants (209 of 213: 106 individual treatment; 103 group treatment) who completed the fourth and last structured treatment session also completed an assessment of

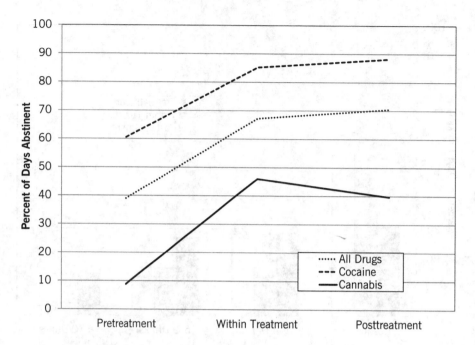

FIGURE 1.4. Percent of days abstinent from drugs during pretreatment, within treatment, and posttreatment for all drug abusers, and separately for cocaine and cannabis abusers.

treatment, rating several aspects of their treatment on 5-point scales (with lower scores reflecting more favorable ratings). Table 1.4 shows clients' end-of-treatment ratings for group and individual conditions and for clients with primary alcohol problems or primary drug problems. Some of the differences, as noted in Table 1.4, are statistically significant.

Overall, clients in both the individual- and the group-treatment conditions rated the program very positively, with mean ratings near the favorable end of the scale (1.42 and 1.56, respectively). Several other aspects of the intervention were also highly rated: quality of service, self-change component, therapists, self-monitoring logs, and the program atmosphere. In fact, with the exception of the length of the treatment and the difficulty of the homework, all mean ratings were positive. With regard to treatment length, group clients were more likely to rate the treatment as being "too little" (mean = 3.55) than individual clients (mean = 3.17), although the mean ratings for this variable suggested that clients in both conditions would have liked the treatment to be longer. Because this study was an RCT, the length of treatment was kept constant. However, in practice the GSC treatment model is flexible and allows for additional sessions. Clients in the group condition also rated the readings and the homework exercises as more useful than clients in the individual condition. One reason this may have occurred is that in the group condition the homework assignments formed the basis of round-robin discussions and, as such, received more attention and talk time because they were discussed by multiple clients. Last, and very important, clients were highly satisfied with being assigned to the group condition (mean = 1.55, with 1 = very satisfied). With regard to the statistically significant differences shown in Table 1.4, they were small in absolute magnitude, and there was no consistent direction of difference.

TABLE 1.4. Clients' End-of-Treatment Ratings of Treatment by Condition (Individual or Group) and by Primary Substance Problem (Alcohol or Drug)

Variable	Treatment condition	
	Individual ($n = 107$) Mean (SD)	Group ($n = 106$) Mean (SD)
Satisfied with treatment (1 = very, 5 = not at all)	1.42 (0.74)[a]	1.56 (0.76)[b]
Quality of service (1 = excellent, 5 = poor)*	1.23 (0.46)[a]	1.43 (0.59)[c]
Program length (1 = too much, 5 = too little)*	3.17 (0.64)[a]	3.55 (0.73)[d]
Satisfied with self-change component (1 = very, 5 = not at all)	1.91 (0.93)[a]	1.84 (0.97)[b]
Satisfied with therapist (1 = very, 5 = not at all)*	1.16 (0.44)[a]	1.42 (0.69)[b]
Readings useful (1 = very, 5 = not at all)*	2.25 (0.99)[e]	1.86 (0.93)[b]
Homework useful (1 = very, 5 = not at all)*	2.03 (0.96)[e]	1.68 (0.89)[d]
Homework difficulty (1 = too easy, 5 = too hard)	2.78 (0.62)[f]	2.86 (0.73)[d]
Self-monitoring useful (1 = very, 5 = not at all)	1.66 (0.83)[e]	1.65 (0.93)[b]
Decisional balance exercise useful (1 = very, 5 = not at all)*	2.23 (0.98)[e]	1.93 (0.89)[b]
Satisfied with program atmosphere (1 = very, 5 = not at all)	1.50 (0.75)[e]	1.69 (0.89)[b]
Program was helpful (1 = very much, 5 = not very much)	1.43 (0.66)[e]	1.52 (0.73)[d]
Recommend program to friend (1 = definitely, 5 = definitely not)	1.23 (0.50)[a]	1.27 (0.61)[g]
Satisfied with being in group (1 = very, 5 = not at all)		1.55 (0.76)[h]

Variable	Primary substance problem	
	Alcohol ($n = 180$) Mean (SD)	Drugs ($n = 33$) Mean (SD)
Satisfied with treatment (1 = very, 5 = not at all)	1.49 (0.76)[h]	1.53 (0.76)[i]
Quality of service (1 = excellent, 5 = poor)	1.34 (0.54)[j]	1.26 (0.51)[k]
Program length (1 = too much, 5 = too little)	3.34 (0.67)[j]	3.44 (0.91)[d]
Satisfied with self-change component (1 = very, 5 = not at all)	1.89 (0.98)[j]	1.81 (0.78)[i]
Satisfied with therapist (1 = very, 5 = not at all)	1.30 (0.60)[h]	1.22 (0.55)[i]
Readings useful (1 = very, 5 = not at all)	2.01 (0.99)[l]	2.34 (0.90)[i]
Homework useful (1 = very, 5 = not at all)	1.80 (0.94)[l]	2.16 (0.92)[i]
Homework difficulty (1 = too easy, 5 = too hard)	2.84 (0.68)[l]	2.71 (0.82)[k]
Self-monitoring useful (1 = very, 5 = not at all)*	1.58 (0.84)[j]	2.06 (0.98)[i]
Decisional balance exercise useful (1 = very, 5 = not at all)	2.09 (0.96)[j]	2.03 (0.90)[i]
Satisfied with program atmosphere (1 = very, 5 = not at all)	1.58 (0.81)[l]	1.66 (0.83)[j]
Program was helpful (1 = very much, 5 = not very much)	1.46 (0.68)[l]	1.53 (0.76)[i]
Recommend program to friend (1 = definitely, 5 = definitely not)	1.25 (0.55)[h]	1.25 (0.62)[i]
Satisfied with being in group (1 = very, 5 = not at all)	1.57 (0.76)[m]	1.47 (0.77)[n]

Note. Ratings made on 5-point scales (1–5) with end points shown for each variable.
[a]n, 106; [b]n, 103; [c]n, 101; [d]n, 102; [e]n, 105; [f]n, 104; [g]n, 100; [h]n, 177; [i]n, 32; [j]n, 176; [k]n, 31; [l]n, 175; [m]n, 81; [n]n, 19;
*$p < .05$, two-tailed independent sample t-tests.

Clients' Evaluations of the GSC Intervention at the 12-Month Follow-Up

At the end of the 12-month follow-up, clients again rated their treatment experiences. Table 1.5 shows clients' evaluations of treatment at the 12-month follow-up for both the group and individual conditions and for clients with primary alcohol and primary drug problems. A total of 230 clients completed the follow-up questionnaires. Similar to their evaluations at the end of treatment, clients' overall evaluations of their treatment at the follow-up were positive, with more than 90% suggesting that the GSC program should continue and over 80% reporting that their substance use was either no longer a problem or less of a problem than before they entered treatment. Interestingly, and consistent with the end-of-treatment evaluations, 42.1% felt that the GSC treatment was not long enough. In this regard, there is substantial evidence that many alcohol and drug abusers with less severe problems show great improvement in brief treatment (e.g., Marijuana Treatment Project Research Group, 2004; Moyer, Finney, Swearingen, & Vergun, 2002; Stephens et al., 2000; Stern, Meredith, Gholson, Gore, & D'Amico, 2007). For example, in a multicenter RCT that compared two 12-session treatments delivered over 12 weeks (12-Step Facilitation and Cognitive-Behavioral Coping Skills) with a 4-session treatment (Motivational Enhancement treatment) delivered over 12 weeks, there were no important differences in outcomes between the treatments (Project MATCH Research Group, 1998). This finding is consistent with other studies showing that a sizeable proportion of individuals with various psychiatric disorders achieve successful outcomes after a few treatment sessions (Wilson, 1999). Thus, although clients in the present study felt that they would have liked more treatment, whether a longer treatment would have yielded better outcomes remains an empirical question. Finally, at the end of follow-up, 82.5% of individual and 81.0% of group clients felt that treatment goals should be self-selected. In addition, 87.7% of individual and 87.1% of group clients said that choosing their own goals was a good thing.

Clients' Evaluations of Group Treatment at Follow-Up

As discussed earlier, the literature shows that when given a choice most clients say they would prefer individual over group therapy. Thus it was decided that at the end of the 12-month follow-up and after all the outcome data had been collected, clients would again be asked to rate their treatment experience, this time including what treatment condition they would have chosen if they had been given a choice at the start of the study. Although it was a retrospective evaluation, significantly more group (38.2%) than individual (5.8%) clients stated at their 12-month follow-up that if given their choice they would have selected group treatment. This suggests that there was a preexisting bias against group therapy that to some extent was lessened by the clients' experience in the groups. At the end of the follow-up, 59.2% of the group clients and 75.6% of all clients still said they would have chosen individual treatment if given a choice. Consistent with the literature, these findings suggest that if group therapy is to be offered, providers need to include pregroup induction procedures to explain the benefits of group therapy and to attend to questions that potential group members may have about group therapy and its effectiveness. Finally, 75.4% of the individual and 65.5% of the group clients said they would prefer to be given the choice between individual and group treatment rather than being assigned to a treatment condition.

TABLE 1.5. Clients' Evaluations of Treatment at the 12-Month Follow-Up by Condition (Individual or Group) and by Primary Substance Problem (Alcohol or Drug)

	Treatment condition	
Question	Individual (IT) ($n = 114$)	Group (GT) ($n = 116$)
Amount of treatment		
% too little	36.3[a]	47.8[b]
% sufficient	62.8	51.3
% too much	0.9	0.9
Drinking status		
% no longer a problem	30.7	31.0
% less of a problem	50.0	52.6
% unchanged	16.7	14.7
% more of a problem	2.6	1.7
Choose own goal		
% good thing	87.7	87.1
% bad thing	4.4	5.2
% no opinion	7.9	7.8
Who should select goal?		
% self-select	82.5	81.0
% therapist select	10.5	12.1
% no opinion	7.0	6.9
Program should continue		
% yes	90.4	93.9[b]
% no	2.6	0.9
% no opinion	7.0	5.2
If assigned to GT, would have participated		
% yes	61.4	
% no	33.3	
% do not know	5.3	
If assigned to IT, would have participated		
% yes		92.2
% no		6.0
% do not know		1.7
If given choice, would have chosen**		
% IT	91.9[c]	59.2[d]
% GT	5.8	38.2
% no opinion	2.3	2.6

(cont.)

TABLE 1.5. *(cont.)*

	Primary substance problem	
Question	Alcohol ($n = 189$)	Drugs ($n = 41$)
Amount of treatment		
% too little	40.1[e]	51.2
% sufficient	58.8	48.8
% too much	1.1	0.0
Drinking status		
% no longer a problem	31.2	29.3
% less of a problem	52.4	46.3
% unchanged	14.8	19.5
% more of a problem	1.6	4.9
Choose own goal		
% good thing	88.9	80.5
% bad thing	3.7	9.8
% no opinion	7.4	9.8
Who should select goal*		
% self-select	86.2	61.0
% therapist select	9.0	22.0
% no opinion	4.8	17.1
Program should continue		
% yes	92.1	92.5[f]
% no	1.6	2.5
% no opinion	6.3	5.0
If assigned to GT, would have participated		
% yes	60.4[g]	66.7[h]
% no	33.3	33.3
% do not know	6.3	0.0
If assigned to IT, would have participated		
% yes	91.4[i]	95.7[j]
% no	7.5	0.0
% do not know	1.1	4.3
If given choice, would have chosen		
% IT	74.4[k]	86.2[l]
% GT	22.6	13.8
% no opinion	3.0	0.0

Note. At the last follow-up (12 months), GT participants were asked, "If you had been assigned to individual treatment rather than group, would you have continued to participate in this study?" and IT clients were asked, "If you had been assigned to group treatment rather than individual, would you have continued to participate in this study?"

[a]n, 113; [b]n, 115; [c]n, 86; [d]n, 76; [e]n, 187; [f]n, 40; [g]n, 96; [h]n, 18; [i]n, 93; [j]n, 23; [k]n, 133; [l]n, 29.
*$p < .01$; **$p < .001$.

Therapists' Evaluation of Clients at the End of Treatment

Another unique aspect of this study was that at the end of the fourth treatment session therapists completed a form evaluating their clients' participation and progress in treatment. Table 1.6 displays therapists' evaluations of clients for group and individual conditions and for clients with primary alcohol and primary drug problems. There were no significant differences between treatment conditions. Only 1 of 13 differences between alcohol and drug clients was statistically significant, with therapists rating alcohol clients as more likely to be on time for sessions than drug clients. What is striking about these evaluations is that irrespective of clients' treatment condition (group vs. individual) or their primary substance abuse problem (alcohol or drug), the therapists' evaluations were uniformly high, reflecting their views that their clients were responsive to treatment, participated actively, and completed their homework assignments.

DISSEMINATION OF THE GSC TREATMENT MODEL: FROM BENCH TO BEDSIDE

We developed the GSC treatment model when we were at the Addiction Research Foundation in Toronto, Canada. As a government-funded agency in a country with government-funded universal health care, the dissemination of effective and efficient treatments was a priority. The story of how the GSC treatment mode was effectively disseminated throughout the province of Ontario, which is the largest province in Canada, has been described in detail elsewhere (Martin, Herie, Turner, & Cunningham, 1998; L. C. Sobell, 1996) but is summarized here as it provides an illustration of the challenges of going from bench to bedside. At the outset of the dissemination effort, we were struck by the fact that although the Addiction Research Foundation was a well-known and internationally respected center for addiction research, evidence-based treatment was not widely used in the community. It was clear that the usual methods of dissemination (e.g., workshops, publications) had not been particularly effective and that, if we wanted to successfully disseminate the GSC treatment model, we would have to think outside the box. In this case, the "box" was the traditional way of attempting to disseminate clinical science, and "outside the box" meant to learn from the experience of others (i.e., business organizations) for which successful dissemination is a matter of survival.

In business, establishing new products requires a substantial and long-term investment in resources (once the product is launched the company must be prepared to respond to demand if sales skyrocket). Failure to obtain buyers for a product can have dire economic consequences. Such research has been described in detail in *Diffusion of Innovations* by Rogers (1995), who is considered the father of dissemination research. Rogers's book was the starting point in developing our efforts to get community treatment providers to adopt the GSC approach.

As described elsewhere (L. C. Sobell, 1996), we successfully partnered with practitioners in the community to disseminate the GSC treatment model. One of the key factors was having a flexible and adaptable product that we could use to train practitioners in the province of Ontario. Before this project, our dissemination efforts typically would have involved offering practitioners a 1-day workshop and handing out treatment materials. In contrast, we engaged in a carefully planned effort that unfolded over time, involving gaining a buy-in from community providers, which brought with it a responsibility on our part to provide continued training and consultation.

TABLE 1.6. Therapists' Evaluations of Clients by Condition (Individual or Group) and by Primary Substance Problem (Alcohol or Drug)

	Treatment condition	
Variable	Individual (*n* = 109) Mean (*SD*)	Group (*n* = 106) Mean (*SD*)
Responsive to treatment	4.48 (0.73)[a]	4.38 (0.79)
Completed homework	4.61 (0.82)	4.67 (0.70)
Participated actively	4.70 (0.59)	4.52 (0.62)
Punctual for sessions	4.60 (0.81)	4.70 (0.57)
Appeared satisfied with sessions	4.53 (0.62)	4.50 (0.62)
Understood homework	4.54 (0.73)	4.72 (0.60)
Appeared ready to change	4.27 (0.93)	4.31 (0.94)
Read handouts	4.73 (0.63)	4.83 (0.47)
Resistant to the treatment program	1.40 (0.81)	1.39 (0.76)
Unresponsive to feedback	1.50 (0.89)	1.40 (0.71)
Worked on self-selected goals	4.63 (0.63)	4.58 (0.80)
Good rapport with therapist	4.60 (0.60)	4.50 (0.56)

	Primary substance problem	
Variable	Alcohol (*n* = 182) Mean (*SD*)	Drugs (*n* = 33) Mean (*SD*)
Responsive to treatment	4.43 (0.75)[b]	4.45 (0.79)
Completed homework	4.65 (0.73)	4.55 (0.91)
Participated actively	4.60 (0.62)	4.67 (0.54)
Got along with others in the group	4.65 (0.53)[c]	4.75 (0.55)[d]
Punctual for sessions*	4.72 (0.55)	4.24 (1.17)
Appeared satisfied with sessions	4.51 (0.62)	4.58 (0.61)
Understood homework	4.62 (0.69)	4.67 (0.60)
Appeared ready to change	4.29 (0.92)	4.27 (1.04)
Read handouts	4.80 (0.52)	4.67 (0.74)
Resistant to the treatment program	1.40 (0.79)	1.39 (0.75)
Unresponsive to feedback	1.48 (0.83)	1.27 (0.67)
Worked on self-selected goals	4.62 (0.69)	4.55 (0.91)
Good rapport with therapist	4.53 (0.59)	4.67 (0.48)

Note. Ratings were made on 5-point scales (1 = *never*, 5 = *always*).
[a]*n*, 108; [b]*n*, 181; [c]*n*, 85, group only; [d]*n*, 20, group only.
*$p < .01$.

Target systems for the treatment were carefully selected through a market analysis and community forums, with the first target system being assessment/referral centers (Martin et al., 1998). Ten workshops were conducted to train center staff in how to conduct GSC treatment in group and individual formats. Of the 42 total assessment/referral centers in the province of Ontario, 39 participated in the training, involving more than 200 staff members.

An important element in creating a favorable response to GSC treatment among community service providers was encouraging them to tailor the procedures to fit their needs. That is, they were encouraged to integrate aspects of the GSC treatment approach that they felt were effective into their existing practices rather than totally discarding one approach for another. Another important element was the provision of ongoing clinical support. A toll-free number was established from our GSC program in Toronto to provide consultation to the field sites. A training videotape demonstrating the GSC intervention was also produced (L. C. Sobell & Sobell, 1995). These efforts resulted in wide-scale adoption of the GSC treatment model throughout the province of Ontario (Martin et al., 1998; L. C. Sobell, 1996).

Our experience in disseminating the GSC treatment model in Ontario has had a lasting influence on our work, including how we have gone about preparing this book. Although we cannot approach the task of writing a book with the same resources, time commitment, or personal involvement that went into the community dissemination effort, we hope that the contents of this book demonstrate a sensitivity to clinicians' and clients' needs and to the context in which cognitive-behavioral group therapy using motivational interviewing is likely to successfully occur.

OVERVIEW OF THIS BOOK

In setting the stage for the remainder of this book, this chapter has reviewed the development of the GSC treatment model and research that influenced its development, compared the GSC treatment model with other cognitive-behavioral therapy for substance use disorders, reviewed the few published RCTs of group versus individual treatment for substance use disorders, and presented the results of the RCT that successfully extended the GSC individual treatment model to a group therapy format.

The remainder of this book presents the details of GSC treatment and how to integrate and implement it in a group setting. It also addresses a plethora of issues and challenges that face therapists who conduct groups (e. g., failure to systematically use group processes, failure to integrate cognitive-behavioral techniques with group processes). Chapter 2, a general overview of motivational interviewing, describes and presents examples of motivational interviewing strategies and techniques and their utility. The strategies and techniques reviewed in Chapter 2 have been an integral part of the GSC treatment model for many years, including the study that compared GSC treatment in a group versus an individual format.

Chapter 3 contains a detailed discussion of how to conduct the GSC assessment, which is the same whether the treatment is delivered in an individual or a group format. This chapter also describes the clinical utility of the assessment measures and instruments that are used in GSC sessions. The therapist dialogues included in Chapter 3 are presented as examples of how topics might be initiated and probed rather than as clinical scripts. Chapters 4 and 5 describe the detailed application of the GSC model to the conduct of individual and group therapy, respectively. Descriptions of each of the four individual treatment sessions and each of the four group treatment sessions include (1) therapist and client handouts, (2) clinical examples, and (3) sample therapist–client dialogues. In addition, both chapters present session outlines for therapists (i.e., objectives, procedures, materials and handouts needed) for each of four individual sessions (Therapist Handouts 4.1–4.4) and each of the four group sessions (Group Therapist Handouts 5.1–5.4). The session outlines for group therapists also include sample round-robin discussions for each group session. Last, Chapter 5 contains a detailed discussion of how to integrate motivational interviewing and cognitive-behavioral strategies and techniques into group therapy using round-robin discussions.

Chapter 6 discusses the importance of group preparation and planning, managing the group, and building group cohesion. This chapter also presents specific examples of how to successfully conduct cognitive-behavioral motivational group therapy using group processes. In this chapter we use two phrases that we feel are key to understanding how to successfully manage groups. The first, *Think Group*, is intended to help group leaders remember that groups have multiple members and that the group itself should be the agent of change. The second phrase, *Music Comes from the Group*, is used to communicate that group therapists can be viewed as conductors and that to achieve high group cohesion, which is related to successful treatment outcomes, the majority of interactions within the group need to come from the members (i.e., the music comes from the group).

Chapters 7 and 8 discuss two central aspects of how to manage groups. Chapter 7 addresses a multitude of structural issues (e.g., composition, attendance, role of cotherapists, breaking eye contact) that are critical for therapists to understand when conducting group therapy. Also included is a brief discussion of the major advantages and disadvantages of conducting group therapy compared with individual therapy. Chapter 8 discusses how to deal with challenging clients and difficult situations in groups. Specific examples for dealing with such situations are provided throughout the chapter.

Chapter 9, the concluding chapter, presents a discussion of the likely place of group psychotherapy in the health care system of the future. This chapter suggests that, as interest in and popularity of group therapy continues to grow, a major challenge will be to ensure that practitioners are competently trained to provide group therapy.

Finally, because the inclusion of clinical materials that could be freely copied and used by clinicians was successfully received in our 1993 book, *Problem Drinkers: Guided Self-Change Treatment* (M. B. Sobel & Sobell, 1993), we have again included a variety of materials that can be reproduced and used by practitioners and, where appropriate, given to clients. These materials include individual and group session outlines, clinical assessment materials, questionnaires, therapist and client handouts, homework exercises, and motivational feedback materials used during both group and individual sessions. With the exception of the group session outlines, all of the assessment and clinical materials can be used when applying the GSC treatment model in either group or individual therapy.

CHAPTER 2

Overview of Motivational Interviewing Strategies and Techniques

There has been considerable interest shown in motivational interviewing (MI), since Miller (1983) initially presented it as an alternative and potentially more effective way of working with problem drinkers, particularly those individuals who may have been perceived as being resistant or in denial.
—BRITT, BLAMPIED, AND HUDSON (2003, p. 193)

[From] humble beginnings two decades ago, MI has been widely adopted and adapted for use with a diverse range of clients.
—ALLSOP (2007, p. 343)

HISTORICAL DEVELOPMENT OF MOTIVATIONAL INTERVIEWING

This chapter provides a general overview of motivational interviewing and its rationale. In the mid-1980s, dissatisfaction with confrontational alcohol treatment approaches, coupled with the conceptualization of motivation as a state (Prochaska & DiClemente, 1982) led William Miller in the United States and Steve Rollnick in the United Kingdom (Miller, 1985; Miller & Rollnick, 1991) to develop motivational interviewing. In their seminal book *Motivational Interviewing*, Miller and Rollnick (1991) noted that there is "no persuasive evidence that aggressive confrontational tactics are even helpful, let alone superior or preferable strategies in the treatment of addictive behavior or other problems" (p. 7). They felt that confrontational approaches, such as insisting that clients label themselves as "alcoholics" or "addicts," served iatrogenically to evoke resistance and could even be counterproductive. For example, individuals who are not severely dependent (e.g., problem drinkers, marijuana abusers, adolescents) may respond to labeling with counterarguing whereby they generate reasons why the label is not applicable to them (Perloff, 2008). In contrast, motivational interviewing does not use labels and deliberately avoids confrontation or other approaches likely to be perceived by the client as judgmental or coercive.

Motivational interviewing has been characterized as a client-centered, directive, noncon-frontational, and nonjudgmental way of interacting with clients that prompts them to give voice to the need for change (Center for Substance Abuse Treatment, 1999; Miller & Rollnick, 2002; Rollnick, Miller, & Butler, 2008). The motivational interviewing strategies and techniques reviewed in this chapter are those that have been an integral part of the GSC treatment model for many years and were used in the study described throughout this book. For clinical guidelines and a detailed discussion of how to use motivational interviewing in a group format, readers are referred to Chapter 6.

Studies comparing motivational interviewing with traditional confrontational treatment approaches for SUDs have found motivational interviewing to result in less resistance, increased compliance, lower dropout rates, better attendance during treatment, and better overall treatment outcomes (Harper & Hardy, 2000; Martino, Carroll, O'Malley, & Rounsaville, 2000; Swanson, Pantalon, & Cohen, 1999).Twenty-five years after its development, motivational interviewing has been evaluated in diverse settings (e.g., health, mental health, medical, health promotion) and with a wide variety of health and mental health problems. These studies, like those for SUDs, have also have found increased compliance, reduced resistance, decreased dropouts, and better treatment outcomes (Britt et al., 2003; Burke, Arkowitz, & Menchola, 2003; Dunn, Deroo, & Rivara, 2001; Knight, McGowan, Dickens, & Bundy, 2006; Miller, 1985, 2005; Miller & Rollnick, 2002; Resnicow et al., 2002; Rollnick & Allison, 2001; Rollnick et al., 2008; Santa Ana, Wolfert, & Nietert, 2007).

Further evidence of the widespread adoption of motivational interviewing is demonstrated by the following figures: (1) the first edition of Miller and Rollnick's book, *Motivational Interviewing: Preparing People to Change Addictive Behavior* (Miller & Rollnick, 1991), sold over 55,000 copies; (2) the second edition (Miller & Rollnick, 2002), according to the publisher (Guilford Press), has as of this writing sold over 180,000 copies and was voted one of the 10 most influential books by *Psychotherapy Networker* readers; and (3) the Motivational Interviewing Network of Trainers (*www.motivationalinterview.org*) reports getting over 41,000 hits per month on their website.

WHAT IS MOTIVATIONAL INTERVIEWING?

Motivational interviewing, an amalgamation of principles and techniques culled from different treatment models and principles of behavior change (e.g., stages of change, Rogerian client-centered therapy, social cognitive learning theory), is a goal-directed, client-centered counseling style. It is designed to elicit intrinsic motivation to change by exploring and resolving a client's ambivalence about changing risky/problem behaviors. Rather than being prescriptive (i.e., telling clients what to do), a motivational interviewing approach uses reflections and other strategies to get clients to verbalize their need to change. Motivational interviewing also helps clients resolve ambivalence by identifying discrepancies between their current behaviors (e.g., continuing to engage in a risky/problem behavior) and their desired goals (e.g., wanting to change a risky/problem behavior) while minimizing resistance. Although motivational interviewing is particularly useful during the early phases of treatment, when resistance is often high, it can be used throughout all phases of treatment, as it is a style conducive to a positive therapeutic relationship.

Ambivalence: A Normal Occurrence

Part of a motivational interviewing approach is recognition by therapists that ambivalence is a normal everyday occurrence, which makes change difficult. Ambivalence is not a reluctance to do something. Rather, it is a conflict about choosing between two courses of action (e.g., continuing to smoke cigarettes vs. quitting; staying in a marriage vs. getting a divorce; doing regular finger pricks to assess one's blood sugar levels vs. not doing them regularly), each of which typically has costs and benefits. In many ways, ambivalence is a battle between conflicting emotions. This is consistent with the Latin origin of the word *ambivalence*, where *ambi-* means *both* and *valence* is derived from *valentia-* meaning *strength*.

Empathy: A Key Element in Motivational Interviewing

Empathy is one of the most important elements of a motivational interviewing approach. An empathic style (1) communicates respect for and acceptance of clients and their feelings, (2) encourages a nonjudgmental, collaborative relationship between the therapist and client, (3) establishes a safe and open environment for the client that is conducive to examining issues and eliciting reasons for change, (4) compliments rather than denigrates, and (5) allows clients to make choices rather than having therapists or practitioners telling them what to do.

The key to expressing empathy is to use reflective listening, in which therapists listen carefully and then reflect back to the client what they think the client has said. By using reflective listening, therapists validate that they understand the client's feelings and concerns (e.g., *"It sounds like you are ambivalent about changing"*). High levels of empathy are associated with positive treatment outcomes for clients with SUDs (Connors, Carroll, DiClemente, Longabaugh, & Donovan, 1997; Miller & Brown, 1997), as well those with psychiatric problems (Horvath & Luborsky, 1993).

Motivational Interviewing:
An Intervention or an Interactional Counseling Style?

In the literature, motivational interviewing has been defined and presented both as an intervention and as an interactional counseling style (e.g., Resnicow et al., 2002). In part, the confusion has arisen from Project MATCH (Heather, 1999; Project MATCH, 1993; Project MATCH Research Group, 1997), a multisite study of treatments for alcohol problems. In Project MATCH a treatment utilizing motivational interviewing was designed as an intervention referred to as Motivational Enhancement Therapy. The first to comment on this were Saunders and Wilkinson (1990), who several years ago said, "Motivational interviewing is not a treatment in itself, but is rather one component in the counseling process" (p. 139). Comments from others, including Miller and Rollnick, support the view that motivational interviewing is an interactional counseling style rather than an intervention: (1) "Rather, it is an *interpersonal style*, not at all restricted to formal counseling settings. It is a subtle balance of directive and client-centered components shaped by a guiding philosophy and understanding of what triggers change" (Rollnick & Miller, 1995, p. 325, emphasis added); (2) "Motivational interviewing has become widely adopted as a *counseling style* for promoting behavior change" (Markland, Ryan, Tobin, & Rollnick, 2005, p. 118, emphasis added); and (3) "Motivational interviewing (MI) is a *counseling style* that has been shown to reduce heavy drinking among college students" (Walters, Vader, Harris, Field, & Jouriles, 2009, p. 64, emphasis added).

Focus and Tone of Motivational Interviewing

In motivational interviewing the focus is on the clients' concerns and beliefs about changing their risky/problem behaviors. A client's ambivalence is explored in a manner that increases motivation to change without eliciting resistance. Motivational interviewing does not attempt to convince or coerce clients into changing. Rather, the intent is to get clients to give voice to the need to change. Using motivational interviewing strategies and techniques, as shown in the following example, allows therapists to guide clients through the change process with clients doing much of the work.

EXAMPLE OF HAVING THE CLIENT GIVE VOICE TO CHANGING

THERAPIST: *"You mentioned that your drinking has started to cause you more problems in the last year, especially with your family. What will happen if you continue to drink over the next year?"*

CLIENT: *"If I don't stop drinking I think it is just a matter of time until my wife and kids leave me."*

The tone of a motivational interviewing approach is empathic, nonjudgmental, nonconfrontational, and supportive, such that clients feel comfortable discussing the good and less good things about their risky/problem behavior(s). Therapists who use a motivational interviewing tone avoid (1) moralizing (e.g., *"You should ... "*), (2) sounding judgmental (e.g., *"You are wrong to think that you can quit by reducing your drinking"*), (3) being stigmatizing (e.g., using labels such as *addict*), and (4) being confrontational (e.g., *"Can't you see that you are going to kill yourself if you don't stop doing drugs?"*).

Content of Motivational Interviewing

While a motivational interviewing style is designed to minimize resistance, the content of motivational interviewing interactions is intended to elicit dialogue and change talk from clients. *Content* relates to what is said. As reflected in the following examples, there are huge differences between a nonmotivational and a motivational way of asking clients about their behavior (i.e., content).

Content reflecting a nonmotivational interviewing style

- *"Do you have a drug problem?"*

- *"Are you an alcoholic?"*

Content reflecting a motivational interviewing style

- *"Do you mind if we talk about your recent drug use?"*

- *"What are the good and less good things about your alcohol use?"*

- *"Why aren't you taking your medication regularly?"*

- *"You need to stop smoking as it is bad for your health."*

- *"If you don't take your insulin regularly you can die."*

- *"What are some of the obstacles you have experienced that have not allowed you to take your medication regularly?"*

- *"It sounds like you are ambivalent about quitting smoking."*

- *"It sounds like you are ambivalent about taking your insulin. What do you think will happen if you don't take it regularly?"*

The nonmotivational questions and comments are closed- or dead-ended (i.e., can be answered in one or two words), confrontational, and sound more like an interrogation. In many cases, nonmotivational questions use labels (e.g., *alcoholic*) and are judgmental (*"Why aren't you taking your insulin?"*). On the other hand, motivational questions, which typically are open-ended, set the stage for clients to provide more information and to establish a dialogue between the client and the therapist.

MOTIVATIONAL INTERVIEWING STRATEGIES AND TECHNIQUES

Several motivational interviewing strategies and techniques are used in GSC treatment, whether delivered in a group or an individual format: asking permission, eliciting change talk, exploring the importance and confidence of changing, asking open-ended questions, employing reflective listening, normalizing, using decisional balancing deploying discrepancies by using the Columbo approach, making statements that support self-efficacy and using the readiness ruler, affirmations, information and feedback, summaries, rolling with resistance, and the therapeutic paradox. The rationale for examples of these motivational interviewing strategies and techniques are discussed next.

Asking Permission

Asking the client's permission to discuss a topic communicates respect for the client. When clients are asked permission to talk about their risky/problem behaviors, they are more likely to be receptive than when they are being lectured to or told to change. Following are some examples of how to ask a client for permission to talk about a risky/problem behavior.

EXAMPLES OF ASKING PERMISSION

- *"Do you mind if we talk about* **[insert risky/problem behavior]***?"*
- *"Can we talk about your* **[insert risky/problem behavior]***?"*
- *"I noticed on your medical history that you have hypertension. Do you mind if we talk about how different lifestyles affect hypertension?"* (Depending on the client, a therapist can mention a particular lifestyle concern, such as diet, exercise, or alcohol use.)

Eliciting Change Talk

Change talk by clients (e.g., stating reasons for the need to change or their intention to change) has been associated with positive outcomes (Apodaca & Longabaugh, 2009; Moyers, Martin, Houck, Christopher, & Tonigan, 2009). The strategy of eliciting change talk contrasts with a therapist's lecturing or telling clients why they should change. Clients' responses to questions intended to elicit change talk usually contain reasons for change that are personally important for them. Eliciting change talk also can address discrepancies between clients' words and actions (e.g., saying that he or she wants to become abstinent but continuing to drink alcohol) in a nonconfrontational manner. One way of doing this, as discussed shortly, is to use a *Columbo approach*. The following are some ways of eliciting change talk.

EXAMPLES OF ELICITING CHANGE TALK

- *"What would you like to see different about your current situation?"*
- *"What makes you think you need to change?"*
- *"What will happen if you don't change?"*
- *"What will be different if you complete your probation?"*
- *"What would be the good things about changing your* **[insert risky/problem behavior]***?"*
- *"What would your life be like 3 years from now if you changed your* **[insert risky/problem behavior]***?"*
- *"Why do you think others are concerned about your* **[insert risky/problem behavior]***?"*

When eliciting change talk with clients who are struggling with changing, therapists need to acknowledge those difficulties using reflective listening and to be supportive of the clients' efforts. For example, a therapist could ask, (1) *"How can I help you get past some of the difficulties you are experiencing?"* or (2) *"If you were to decide to change, what would you have to do to make it happen?"* When clients have expressed little desire to or intention of changing, a therapist can place emphasis on building motivation for change. This can be accomplished, as shown in the following examples by asking clients about extreme outcomes or by telescoping present behavior into the future.

ADDITIONAL EXAMPLES OF ELICITING CHANGE TALK

- *"Suppose you don't change, what is the* **worst** *thing that might happen?"*
- *"What is the* **best** *thing you could imagine that could result from changing?"*
- *"If you make changes, how would your life be different from what it is today?"*
- *"How would you like things to turn out for you in 2 or 3 years?"*

Open-Ended Questions

Open-ended questions are a standard and important feature of a motivational interviewing approach. When therapists use open-ended questions, it allows a richer, deeper conversation that flows and builds empathy with clients. In contrast, multiple back-to-back closed or dead-ended questions can feel like an interrogation (e.g., *"How often do you use cocaine?"; "How many years have you had an alcohol problem?"; "How many times have you been arrested?"*). Open-ended questions also encourage clients to do most of the talking while the therapist listens and responds with reflections or summary statements. In the following examples, note how each question is designed to elicit a conversation from the client (i.e., it would be difficult for the client to respond with a very short answer).

EXAMPLES OF OPEN-ENDED QUESTIONS

- *"Tell me what you like about your* **[insert risky/problem behavior]**.*"*
- *"What's happened since our last session?"*
- *"What makes you think it might be time for a change?"*
- *"What brought you here today?"*
- *"What happens when you act that way?"*
- *"How were you able to not use* **[insert substance]** *for* **[insert time frame]***?"*
- *"Tell me more about when this first began."*
- *"What's different for you this time?"*
- *"What was that like for you?"*
- *"What's different about quitting this time?"*

Reflective Listening

In motivational interviewing, reflective listening is the primary way of responding to clients and building empathy. It involves listening carefully to clients and then reflecting back to them a reasonable guess about what they are saying; in other words, it is like forming and testing a hypothesis. Essentially, the therapist is paraphrasing the clients' comments back to them (e.g., *"It sounds like you have a lot of concerns about how your smoking is affecting your health"*). Reflective listening can also be used with open-ended questions to get clients to state their arguments for change (e.g., *"So, on the one hand you are saying that you want to leave your husband, and yet on the other hand, you are worrying about hurting his feelings by ending the relationship. That must be difficult for you. How do you imagine the two of you would feel in another 3 years if things don't change?"*). Reflections also validate what clients are feeling and communicate that the therapist understands what the client has said (i.e., *"It sounds like you are feeling upset at not getting the job"*).When therapists' reflections are correct, clients usually respond affirmatively. If the guess is wrong (e.g., *"It sounds like you don't want to quit smoking at this time"*), clients usually quickly disconfirm the hypothesis (e.g., *"No, I do want to quit, but I am very dependent and am concerned about withdrawal and weight gain"*). The following are some generic and specific ways of phrasing reflections.

EXAMPLES OF GENERIC REFLECTIONS

- *"***It sounds** like … *"*
- *"What* **I hear you saying** … *"*

- *"So on the one hand* **it sounds** like … and, yet on the other hand … "
- **"It seems** as if … "
- **"I get the sense** that … "
- **"It feels** as though … "

EXAMPLES OF REFLECTIONS FOCUSED ON A SPECIFIC PROBLEM OR ISSUE

- **"It sounds like you** recently became concerned about your **[insert risky/problem behavior]**.*"*
- **"It sounds like your [insert risky/problem behavior]** *has been one way for you to* **[insert function of risky/problem behavior]**.*"*
- **"I get the sense that** you are wanting to change, and you have concerns about your **[insert risky/problem behavior]**.*"*
- **"What I hear you saying is** that your **[insert risky/problem behavior]** *is really not much of a problem right now. What you do think it might take for you to change in the future?"*
- **"I get the feeling** there is a lot of pressure on you to change, but you are not sure you can do it because of past difficulties quitting/changing."

Normalizing

Normalizing is used to communicate that having difficulties changing is not uncommon and that ambivalence is normal. Normalizing is not intended to make clients feel comfortable with not changing. Rather, it is intended to help clients understand that others have had difficulty changing and that they are not alone. The following are some examples of normalizing.

EXAMPLES OF NORMALIZING

- *"A lot of people are concerned about changing their* **[insert risky/problem behavior]**.*"*
- *"Most people report both good and less good things about their* **[insert risky/problem behavior]**.*"*
- *"Many people report feeling like you do. They want to change their* **[insert risky/problem behavior]** *but find it difficult."*
- *"That is not unusual, many people report having made several previous quit attempts."*
- *"A lot of people are concerned about gaining weight when quitting smoking."*

Decisional Balancing

Decisional balancing strategies can be used any time throughout treatment as a way of helping clients recognize and understand their ambivalence. One way to start is to give clients a decisional balance exercise (see Client Handout 3.1) at the assessment session and ask them to bring the completed exercise to their first session. The decisional balance exercise, described in more detail in Chapters 4 and 5, asks clients to evaluate their current behaviors by concurrently looking at the good and less good things about changing and about not changing. The goals of using a decisional balance exercise are twofold: First, to help clients recognize that they get some benefits from their risky/problem behavior and, second, to help them recognize that there will be some costs to changing their behavior. Talking with clients about the good and less good things in their decisional balance exercise can help them to understand their ambivalence about changing and increase their motivation to change. However, rather than having therapists read over the form and ask clients questions, it is better for therapists to ask clients to discuss what they listed for the costs and benefits. This then provides an opportunity for the therapist to reflect and summarize the content back to the client and to elicit change talk (e.g., "Given everything we have talked about, where do you go from here?").

Therapists can also verbally conduct a decisional balance exercise with clients by asking them in an open-ended fashion to describe the good and less good things about their risky/problem behavior and about changing their behavior. For example, a therapist might say, *What are some of the good things about your* [insert risky/problem behavior]*? [Client answers.] Okay, on the flip side, what are some of the less good things about your* [insert risky/problem behavior]*?"* After this discussion, therapists can use a reflective summary statement that includes the clients' statements about the good and less good things with the intent of having clients recognize and discuss their ambivalence about changing.

The Columbo Approach

The Columbo approach takes its name from the behavior demonstrated by Peter Falk, who starred in the 1970s television series *Columbo*. It can be characterized as a way of gently deploying discrepancies to clients. Basically, clients are asked to help therapists make sense of or understand the discrepant information. The Columbo approach is implemented as a curious inquiry about discrepant behaviors without being judgmental. By juxtaposing in a nonconfrontational manner information that is contradictory, the client is made aware of discrepancies in a way that minimizes defensiveness or resistance. The following are some examples of Columbo-like statements.

EXAMPLES OF HOW TO USE THE COLUMBO APPROACH WITH CLIENTS

- *"On the one hand, you're coughing and are out of breath, and, on the other hand, you are saying cigarettes are not causing you any problems. What do you think is causing your breathing difficulties?"*

- *"Help me to understand: On the one hand, you say you want to live to see your 12-year-old daughter grow up and go to college, and yet you won't take the medication your doctor prescribed for your diabetes. How will that help you live to see your daughter grow up?"*

- *"Help me to understand: On the one hand, I hear you say you are worried about retaining custody of your children, and yet, on the other hand, you are telling me that you are occasionally using crack with your boyfriend. I am wondering how keeping custody of your children fits with your cocaine use."*

Supporting Self-Efficacy

Many clients in treatment have low confidence in their ability to change. Because high self-efficacy is associated with better outcomes, it is important to find ways to increase clients' self-efficacy (reviewed in Witkiewitz & Marlatt, 2004). One way therapists can increase clients' self-confidence or self-efficacy is to elicit and support talk about changes clients have made in the past. Another way to increase self-efficacy is using scaling techniques (e.g., readiness ruler, importance and confidence ratings related to goal choice). For example, when using a readiness ruler, if a client's readiness to change goes from a lower number (past) to a higher number (now), therapists can then ask how the person was able to do that and how he or she feels about the change. Following are some examples of how to elicit statements from clients that are likely to increase their self-confidence.

EXAMPLES OF STATEMENTS SUPPORTING SELF-EFFICACY

- *"It seems you've been working hard to quit smoking. That is different than before. How have you been able to do that?"* Follow up by asking, *"How do you feel about this change?"*

- *"Last week you were not sure you could go one day without using cocaine. How were you able to avoid using this past week?"*

- *"So even though you have not been abstinent every day this past week, you have managed to cut your drinking down significantly. How were you able to do that?"* Follow up by asking, *"How do you feel about this?"*

- *"Based on your self-monitoring logs, you have not been using cannabis daily. In fact, you only used one day last week. How were you able to do that?"* Follow up by asking, *"How do you feel about the change?"*

- *"Quitting cocaine seems to be presenting a pretty big challenge to you, but at the assessment you mentioned that 3 years ago you were able to stop on your own for 9 months. How did you do that? What does that tell you about how you can handle what you are facing now?"*

Readiness Ruler

Assessing readiness to change is a critical aspect of motivational interviewing. Motivation, which is considered a state and not a trait, is not static and thus can change from day to day. Clients enter treatment at different levels of motivation or readiness to change (e.g., not ready, ambivalent, ready). The concept of readiness to change is an outgrowth of the stages of change model that conceptualizes individuals as being at different stages of readiness when entering treatment (Heather, Smailes, & Cassidy, 2008). A simple and quick way to evaluate readiness is to use a readiness ruler (Rollnick et al., 2008), a scaling strategy that conceptualizes readiness or motivation to change along a continuum. Using the readiness ruler, clients are asked to give voice to how ready they are to change on a 10-point scale, where 1 = *definitely not ready to change* and 10 = *definitely ready to change*. A readiness ruler allows therapists to immediately know their clients' level of motivation for change. Depending on where the client is, the subsequent conversation will take different directions. For example, with clients who choose a low number (e.g., 1 to 4), therapists can ask, *"What would have to happen for you to go from a 3 to a 5?"* The readiness ruler can also help clients give voice to how they have changed, what they need to do to change further, and how they feel about changing (D'Onofrio, Bernstein, & Rollnick, 1996). The following example demonstrates how to use a readiness ruler.

EXAMPLE OF USING THE READINESS RULER

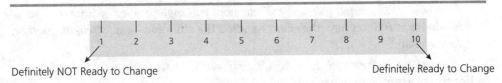

Definitely NOT Ready to Change   Definitely Ready to Change

THERAPIST: *"On a scale from 1 to 10, where 1 is definitely not ready to change and 10 is definitely ready to change, what number best reflects how ready you are at the present time to change your* **[insert risky/problem behavior]***?"*

CLIENT: *"Seven."*

THERAPIST: *"On this same scale, where were you 6 months ago?"*

CLIENT: *"Two."*

THERAPIST: *"So it sounds like you went from not being ready to change your* **[insert risky/problem behavior]** *to thinking about changing. How did you go from a 2 six months ago to a 7 now?"*

After the client answers, the therapist can follow up and ask, *"How do you feel about making those changes?"* and *"What would it take to move a bit higher on the scale?"*

Although they are few in number, some clients will report a decrease in their readiness to change over time. In such cases, the therapist's interaction can focus on identifying ways to increase readiness. The following is an example of a client who reports decreasing his or her readiness to change over time: *"So 6 months ago you were a 5 and today you say you are at a 2. It sounds like you went from being ambivalent about changing your* [insert risky/problem behavior] *to no longer feeling you need to change your* [insert risky/problem behavior]. *What would have to happen to get you to back to where you were 6 months ago?"*

Affirmations

Affirmations are statements made by therapists in response to what clients have said and are intended to recognize clients' strengths, successes, and efforts to change. Affirmative responses and supportive statements by therapists verify and acknowledge clients' behavior changes, as well as attempts to change. For affirmations to help to increase clients' confidence in their ability to change, they need to sound sincere, not ingratiating (e.g., *"Wow, that's incredible!"* or *"That's great, I knew you could do it!"*). The following are some examples of affirmative statements.

EXAMPLES OF HOW TO FRAME AFFIRMATIVE STATEMENTS

- *"Your commitment really shows by* **[insert a reflection about what the client is doing]**.*"*
- *"You showed a lot of* **[insert what best describes the client's behavior—*strength, courage, determination*]** *by doing that."*
- *"It's clear by your behavior that you're really trying to change your* **[insert risky/problem behavior]**.*"*
- *"By the way you reported handling the situation, you showed a lot of* **[insert descriptive label that reflects how the client handled the situation—e.g., *strength, courage, determination*]**.*"*
- *"Despite all the obstacles you have been facing, you still have refrained from engaging in* **[insert risky/problem behavior]**.*"*
- *"In spite of what happened last week, coming here today reflects that you're concerned about changing your* **[insert risky/problem behavior]**.*"*

Information and Feedback

A frequently used motivational interviewing strategy is providing information or feedback to clients. This is a valuable technique because clients often lack information with which to make informed decisions or have wrong information. Traditionally, therapists and other health care practitioners have encouraged clients to quit or change behaviors using what has been termed *simple advice* (e.g., *"If you continue using you are going to have* **[insert health consequence]**.*"*). The reason simple advice does not work well is that most people do not like being *told what to do*. Rather, most individuals prefer being given a choice in making decisions, particularly when considering changing risky/problem behaviors.

How information is presented can also affect how it is received. Presenting information and feedback in a neutral, nonjudgmental, sensitive manner minimizes resistance and empowers people to make better informed decisions about stopping or changing a risky/problem behavior. One way to provide feedback, for example, is to allow people to evaluate their behavior in relation to national norms (e.g., % of men and women drinking at different levels; % of the population using cannabis last year). Client Handouts 4.1 and 4.2 in Chapter 4 contain examples of how we present such feedback to clients as part of the GSC treatment. Information about health risks is another type of feedback that can be presented to clients (e.g., risk of different cancers related to drinking levels) to increase their motivation to change. Presenting feedback in a motivational manner, as shown in Client Handouts 4.1 and 4.2, allows clients to evaluate the feedback for personal relevance (*"I drink as much as my friends, but maybe we're all drinking more than we should"*).

Whenever possible, materials should be presented with a focus on the positives of changing. An excellent example of positive information that can be provided involves the short-term and long-term health benefits that can accrue from stopping smoking. The figures in Table 2.1 presents information taken from the Centers for Disease Control and Prevention Web page (*www.cdc.gov/tobacco/data_statistics/fact_sheets/cessation/quitting/#benefits*) showing the many health benefits that can derive from quitting smoking. For example, within 20 minutes of quitting smoking, a smoker's body begins a series of changes, starting with an immediate decrease in blood pressure. At 15 years after quitting, the risk of coronary heart disease is the same as that of a nonsmoker. The advantage of providing smokers with such information is that those who have smoked for years often think that they have ruined their health and will receive few, if any, benefits from stopping. To the contrary, as reflected in Table 2.1, the benefits from stopping smoking are dramatic and start right away. Thus, if therapists provide smokers with this information, they can correct this misperception, which in turn might help motivate them to consider quitting. In this regard, therapists can ask current smokers, *"What do you know about the benefits of quitting smoking?"* and follow up by asking permission to talk about the client's smoking (*"Do you mind if we spend a few minutes talking about some of the short-term and long-term benefits of quitting?"*). Giving smokers a pamphlet that outlines the benefits in Table 2.1 might also be helpful.

Remember that some clients will not want information. When therapists use scare tactics, lecture, moralize, or warn of disastrous consequences, they are acting in a way that is contrary to a positive therapeutic relationship. A preferred approach would be to acknowledge the client's position and say something like, *"Okay, perhaps at some future time we could come back to this."* The following are some examples of how to provide information or feedback. It often is helpful to start by asking the client's permission to talk about the behavior.

TABLE 2.1. Benefits of Quitting Smoking Timeline

Quitting smoking can help smokers be healthier and live longer, no matter how old they are when they quit. As described by the Centers for Disease Control and Prevention, the following are some of the many benefits of quitting smoking:

- Smoking cessation lowers the risk for lung and other types of cancer.
- Smoking cessation reduces the risk for coronary heart disease, stroke, and peripheral vascular disease.
- Smoking cessation reduces respiratory symptoms, such as coughing, wheezing, and shortness of breath. The rate of decline in lung function is slower among persons who quit smoking.
- Smoking cessation reduces the risk of developing chronic obstructive pulmonary disease, one of the leading causes of death in the United States.
- Smoking cessation by women during their reproductive years reduces the risk for infertility. Women who stop smoking during pregnancy also reduce their risk of having a low birthweight baby.

Benefits of Quitting Smoking Timeline

Within 20 minutes after smokers have their last cigarette, their bodies begin a series of changes that continue for years. Below is a timeline of benefits of quitting smoking as described by the Centers for Disease Control and Prevention.

20 minutes after quitting: Your heart rate and blood pressure drop.

12 hours after quitting: The carbon monoxide level in your blood drops to normal.

2 weeks–3 months after quitting: Your circulation improves and your lung function increases.

1–9 months after quitting: Coughing and shortness of breath decrease.

1 year after quitting: The excess risk of coronary heart disease is half that of a smoker.

5 years after quitting: Your stroke risk is reduced to that of a nonsmoker 5–15 years after quitting.

10 years after quitting: Your lung cancer death rate is about half that of a person who continues to smoke. The risk of cancer of the mouth, throat, esophagus, bladder, kidney, and pancreas decrease.

15 years after quitting: The risk of coronary heart disease is the same as a nonsmoker.

Note. From the Centers for Disease Control and Prevention (*www.cdc.gov/tobacco/data_statistics/fact_sheets/cessation/quitting/#benefits*).

EXAMPLES OF PROVIDING INFORMATION AND FEEDBACK

SUGGESTED WAYS TO PROVIDE INFORMATION IN A MOTIVATIONAL INTERVIEWING MANNER WITH A CLIENT WHO DRINKS ALCOHOL AT RISK LEVELS AND HAS HYPERTENSION

- *"I noticed on your medical history form that you indicated that you are taking medications for hypertension. Do you mind if we spend a few minutes talking about how alcohol use affects your hypertension?"* **[Can insert any risky/problem behavior here.]**

  [Followed by] *"What do you know about how your alcohol use* **[can insert any risky/problem behavior here]** *affects your hypertension* **[can insert whatever the risky/problem behavior might affect; e.g., health issue]***?"*

  [Followed by] *"Are you interested in learning more about how your drinking* **[insert risky/problem behavior; e.g., alcohol use]** *affects your hypertension?"*

  After the foregoing dialogue, clients can be provided with relevant materials related to changing their risky/problem behavior or what effects it has on other aspects of their lives.

- *"If you like I have some pamphlets about how alcohol can affect hypertension* **[insert health problem]** *that you can read and we can discuss at the next session."*

ADDITIONAL EXAMPLES OF PROVIDING INFORMATION TO CLIENTS IN A MOTIVATIONAL INTERVIEWING MANNER

- *"What do you know about the laws in* **[insert name of state]** *and what will happen if you get a* **second drunk driving arrest***?"* [Client answers: *"I think the legal limit is .08."*] *"What do you know about how many drinks it takes to get to this level?"*

- *"So you said you are* **concerned about gaining weight if you stop smoking***. How much do you think the average person gains in the first year after quitting?"*

- *"I've taken the information about your drinking that you provided at the assessment and calculated what you reported drinking per week on average, and it is shown on this form along with graphs showing levels of drinking in the general population. Where do you fit in?"* [see Chapter 4, Client Handout 4.1]

- *"On one of the questionnaires you filled out, the Drug Abuse Screening Test, you scored a 7. This form shows how scores on that questionnaire are related to drug problem severity. Where do you fit in?"* [see Chapter 4, Client Handout 4.2]

The National Institute on Alcohol Abuse and Alcoholism has a website, Rethinking Drinking Alcohol and Your Health, that readers can use to prepare different types of feedback for their clients in relation to alcohol use (*rethinkingdrinking.niaaa.nih.gov*).

Summary Statements

Therapists can judiciously use summary statements to reinforce what clients have said. Such statements can be used to reflect ambivalence, to move clients on to another topic, or to expand the ongoing discussion. Summaries require that therapists listen very carefully to what clients have said throughout the session. In addition, they are a good way to transition a talkative client to the next topic or to end a session (i.e., offer a summary of the entire session). The following are examples of summary statements.

EXAMPLES OF DIFFERENT SUMMARY STATEMENTS

- *"It sounds like when you started using cocaine there were many positives. Now, however, it sounds like the costs and your increased use, coupled with your girlfriend's complaints, have you thinking about quitting. What will your life be like if you do stop?"*

- *"It sounds like you are concerned about your cocaine use because it is costing you a lot of money and there is a chance you could end up in jail. You also said quitting will probably mean not associating with your friends anymore. That doesn't sound like an easy choice."*

- *"Over the past 3 months you have been talking about stopping using crack, and it seems that just recently you have started to recognize that the less good things about your use are outweighing the good things. That, coupled with your girlfriend leaving you because you continued to use crack, makes it easy to understand why you are now committed to not using crack anymore."*

Rolling with Resistance

In a therapeutic relationship, resistance occurs when two sets of values or goals are in opposition. The therapist wants one thing to happen (e.g., the client to change), and the client wants another thing to happen (e.g., the client feels that there is no need to change). Reluctance to change is natural and understandable, particularly for individuals who do not see themselves as needing to change. Motivational interviewing suggests that a therapist's response to a client's resistance can largely determine the person's subsequent response (Moyers & Rollnick, 2002).

Usually resistance is easy to recognize. When the therapeutic interaction does not feel good, particularly with clients who present as being coerced or say they are not ready to change, this is a signal for therapists to change strategies and use a motivational interviewing approach. This approach recognizes that therapists have a *choice*—to increase resistance or to roll with resistance. When a client is being resistant and the therapist responds by arguing more strongly, the client is likely to get defensive. Such interactions can weaken or destroy the therapeutic relationship, and they are also counterproductive. Such counterproductive responses have been labeled as a *righting reflex*, by which therapists attempt to make things *better* or *set things right* by prescribing or telling clients what to do (e.g., *"If you don't take your insulin you will develop serious health problems which can kill you"* or *"You need to stop smoking cigarettes because they cause cancer and heart attacks and will take years off your life"*).

A motivational interviewing approach offers an alternative of rolling with resistance rather than being confrontational. This approach suggests that therapists leave their agendas at the doorstep and roll with resistance by reflecting the client's situation. Usually this involves acknowledging that the client is not ready to commit to change or to even discussing change. When a therapist responds with reflective statements, this conveys to clients that their therapist understands them. It also avoids arguments when clients are resistive.

The following is an example of using motivational interviewing in a group with one person who is angry due to feeling coerced to attend treatment. In this and similar cases, the group leaders need to reduce resistance by avoiding the use of statements that will increase anger or defensiveness. One way a group leader can do this is by reflecting the person's frustration or anger and then asking the group to provide some alternative strategies for dealing with the current situation. Ultimately, by dealing with resistance, therapists will be more likely to encourage group members to continue in treatment and participate in the group.

EXAMPLE OF DEALING WITH RESISTANCE IN A GROUP

BILL: *"It's enough to be forced to be here, but don't expect me to participate."*

GROUP LEADER: *"Bill, when you say that you're forced to come here, can you tell us what you mean?"*

BILL: *"I came to group because my wife said she would leave me. That's the only reason I'm here, so I'm not happy."*

Group leaders' focus: The following question is intended to get others to comment about having had similar feelings (e.g., being forced to do something, or that they were in treatment largely to satisfy someone else):

> *"Who else in the group can identify with how Bill is feeling and share how they have handled similar situations?"*

After the group responds, one of the group leaders can say:

> *"So several of you have said you've felt somewhat coerced coming here, but most of you have also said you chose to come because it was better than the alternative, such as going to jail or making relationships worse. In what other areas of your lives do you have concerns about having limited choices?"*

Although the above reflection recognizes that others feel the way Bill does (i.e., being forced to attend the group), it also points out that coming to group was their *choice*. The leader's next question (summarizing members' different responses) is intended to get the group talking about limited choices while broadening the topic to deal with limited choice situations generally. This is intended to reduce affect caused by the original topic and to minimize resistance.

> *"So it sounds like there are many situations in life in which choice is an issue, and there will be times when people choose to do something they don't really like because that is the best choice available to them."*

At the end of group, when everyone comments about what stood out, one of the group leaders might offer the following comment in regard to the preceding dialogue:

> *"So, we have heard today that some group members initially felt coerced by others to be here. However, several members also said sometimes people have to choose between two options they don't like, and that involves picking the one that has the fewest negative consequences."*

Therapeutic Paradox

For clients who have been coming to treatment for some time but have made little progress, paradoxical statements can be used in an effort to get them to argue for the importance of changing. It is important to recognize, however, that the use of therapeutic paradoxes involves some risk (i.e., a client could agree with the paradoxical statement rather than arguing for the importance of change). Paradoxical statements are purposely phrased so that they are perceived by clients as unexpected contradictions on the part of the therapist. For example, a therapist might say, *"Bill, I know you have been coming to treatment for two months, but you are still drinking heavily. Maybe now is not the right time to change?"* In making such a statement, it is important to sound genuine and not sarcastic. The intent is that clients, upon hearing such statements, will seek to correct them by arguing for change. Thus a client might respond, *"No, I know I need to change, it's just tough putting it into practice."* If this occurs, subsequent conversations can focus on identifying the reasons that progress has been slow.

In addition, paradoxical statements could have a negative effect on some clients (e.g., clients with low self-efficacy). Thus we recommend using them only, if at all, late in treatment for clients who are not making changes. For example, they could be used with clients who have been attending sessions regularly but have not made any progress toward changing the risky/problem behavior for which they sought treatment.

When using the therapeutic paradox, therapists should be prepared for some clients to decide they do not want to change. In such cases, reasons for not being ready to change or not seeing a need to change can be discussed. If a client feels strongly that the time is not right for change or that change is not possible, it might be suggested that the client take a *time out* from treatment. When this is done, we tell clients that we will call them in a few weeks to touch base with them and see if they want to resume treatment. The following are some examples of statements that can be used to create a therapeutic paradox with clients.

EXAMPLES OF STATEMENTS TO CREATE A THERAPEUTIC PARADOX

- *"Maybe now is not the right time for you to change."*
- *"Mary, you've been continuing to* **[insert risky/problem behavior]**, *and yet you say that you want to* **[insert the behavior the person wants to change—e.g., get your children back; get your driver's license returned; not have your spouse leave]**. *Maybe this is not a good time to try and make those changes."*
- *"So it sounds like you have a lot going on with trying to balance a career and family, and these priorities are competing with treatment at this time. Maybe taking a break from treatment might be helpful."*

SUMMARY

Motivational interviewing is many things, but first and foremost it is a counseling style that works well with many clients—in particular, with those who are ambivalent about changing their behavior. Motivational interviewing is used to build rapport and help clients explore and resolve their ambivalence about changing. Motivational interviewing is conducted in a manner likely to increase a client's motivation to change while minimizing resistance. A major goal of motivational interviewing is for clients to provide the arguments for change (i.e., *give voice*) rather than being told to change by their therapists. Use of motivational interviewing strategies and techniques creates a respectful and empowering interaction wherein clients come to understand their behavior and its motivation and decide upon actions to resolve ambivalence. Simply put, what therapists say (i.e., *content*) and how they say it (i.e., *style*) can have a powerful effect on influencing clients' motivation to consider changing. Although initially developed to treat alcohol abusers, motivational interviewing has become "widely adopted and adapted for use with a diverse range of clients" (Allsop, 2007, p. 343) across many health and mental health fields.

CHAPTER 3

Assessment

A Running Start for Treatment

> The assessment not only gathers data but also provides the start
> of an accelerated treatment process.
> —M. B. SOBELL AND SOBELL (1993a, p. 52)

This chapter presents a detailed discussion of how to conduct the GSC assessment and of the clinical utility of the assessment measures and instruments that are used in the GSC individual and group interventions. The assessment interview gathers information that helps inform the subsequent treatment and constitutes the start of the therapeutic relationship. When clients are asked to provide detailed information about themselves and their problems, we have found that many start to understand their problems and think of plans for how to deal with them. In other words, the assessment process itself may be sufficient to instigate behavior change or at least to catalyze the change process (Clifford, Maisto, & Davis, 2007; Epstein et al., 2005). It is for this reason that in our earlier book on GSC treatment (M. B. Sobell & Sobell, 1993a) we described the assessment as providing a "running start" (p. 57) for treatment. The use of the assessment measures and questionnaires can be modified to fit individual clients or program needs.

USING A MOTIVATIONAL INTERVIEWING APPROACH
TO START THE ASSESSMENT

The assessment begins with a dialogue that is motivational in nature and is intended to express empathy and establish rapport. This, in turn, facilitates the development of a positive therapeutic relationship that is intended to enhance and maintain the client's motivation to change. As reflected in the clinical examples that follow, rather than launching into an interrogation, the therapist uses open-ended questions to encourage clients to discuss why they entered treatment and what they hope to achieve. After this, the GSC treatment program, which helps people help themselves, is briefly described. The assessment then proceeds with collecting background data and information related to the problem for which clients are seeking treatment. Some of the information collected at assessment is then used in subsequent GSC sessions to provide personalized feedback to clients about their alcohol and drug use.

For many clients, especially if their problems are not severe, their participation in the assessment marks the first time they have given serious thought to their problems and what it will take to change their behavior. Consequently, two goals are to make sure that clients feel understood and that they will return for their first session. Suggestions about how to accomplish those goals are contained in sample clinical dialogues that are included throughout this chapter. It should be emphasized, however, that these dialogues are presented as suggestions and examples of how topics might be initiated and probed rather than as clinical scripts.

As mentioned, to foster development of the therapeutic relationship, it is helpful before launching into data collection to have a short discussion with clients about why they are seeking treatment and what their expectations are and to provide them with a description of the treatment program. Following is a sample of what a therapist might say to a client at the start of the assessment.

> *"Before we start, I want to tell you about what we'll be doing today. Today's session will take about 2 hours. We will be talking about many things, such as what brought you to treatment, what you expect to get from treatment, and how you might go about changing your* [insert what brought the person to treatment; e.g., alcohol or drug use]. *Near the end of the assessment I will be asking you to complete some forms, which will be used over the next few sessions to provide you information about your* [insert what brought the person to treatment; e.g., your alcohol or drug use]."

After a brief introduction like the preceding, and actively listening to the client's response, we recommend that therapists provide clients with a brief description or overview of the treatment program in which the client will be participating. The following sample overview provided by the therapist would be the same for GSC treatment delivered in either an individual or a group format. Chapter 5 presents additional information given to clients who will be participating in the group version of the GSC treatment.

> *"The Guided Self-Change treatment program is designed to help you guide your own treatment. You will learn how to use a problem-solving approach to deal with your alcohol or drug use. We are going to ask you to complete some readings and homework exercises and to self-monitor your alcohol and drug use. When people work on things outside of their sessions, it helps accelerate their change. For that reason, it is important to do the assigned homework exercises. The program consists of four semistructured sessions plus today's assessment. In the fourth session, we'll review your progress, and you can decide at that time whether you would like more sessions. One month after your last session, I'll call to see how you are doing. Do you have any questions?"*

ASSESSMENT MEASURES AND QUESTIONNAIRES: DESCRIPTION AND UTILITY

The remainder of this chapter describes in detail the measures and questionnaires used in the GSC group and individual interventions and their utility. Table 3.1 contains a list of the measures and questionnaires used in the individual and group GSC sessions. Most standard assess-

TABLE 3.1. Measures and Questionnaires Used in GSC Treatment for Individual and Group Therapy

- *Drug Use History Questionnaire (DUHQ):* Assesses lifetime and recent drug use.
- *Timeline Followback (TLFB):* Assesses daily substance use prior to treatment.
- *Alcohol Use Disorders Identification Test (AUDIT):* 10-item scale that assesses recent and past alcohol use, consequences, and problem severity.
- *Drug Abuse Screening Test (DAST-10):* 10-item scale that assesses drug use consequences and problem severity over the preceding year.
- *Brief Situational Confidence Questionnaire (BSCQ):* Assesses a client's confidence (i.e., self-efficacy) in his or her ability to resist drinking heavily or using drugs on a scale ranging from 0% (*not at all confident*) to 100% (*very confident*) for eight high-risk situations.
- *Readiness ruler:* Assesses ambivalence and readiness to change.
- *Where Are You Now Scale:* Assesses clients' subjective evaluations of the severity of the problems for which they are seeking treatment.
- *Goal statements:* Allows clients to have a choice in selecting goals and assesses clients' ratings of the importance of their goals and their confidence that they will achieve their goals.
- *Self-monitoring logs:* Clients record various aspects of their substance use (e.g., daily use, urges, situations in which use occurred, thoughts when using), which allows them to report and talk honestly about their substance use throughout treatment.

ment forms used in cognitive-behavioral interventions collect basic demographic data (e.g., age, education, gender) and problem history information. In this regard, the GSC treatment model uses a core assessment questionnaire that collects basic demographic data (e.g., age, education, gender, employment, marital status) and substance use history data (e.g., number of years alcohol or drugs have been a problem, frequency and magnitude of use, alcohol and drug consequences, past change attempts).

Alcohol Use Disorders Identification Test

The Alcohol Use Disorders Identification Test (AUDIT), a 10-item psychometrically sound scale (Appendix A) developed by the World Health Organization, assesses recent and past alcohol use, consequences, and problem severity (Reinert & Allen, 2007). Scores range from 0 to 40, with a score of 8 or more being suggestive of an alcohol problem. The AUDIT is able to detect problem drinkers along a continuum from mild to moderate to severe. As is discussed in Chapter 4, AUDIT scores are used in Session 1 to provide personalized feedback to clients about the seriousness of their alcohol use prior to treatment (see the last page of Client Handout 4.1).

Drug Abuse Screening Test

The Drug Abuse Screening Test (DAST-10; Appendix B) is a 10-item psychometrically sound scale similar to the AUDIT in that it assesses drug consequences and problem severity over the previous year (Gavin, Ross, & Skinner, 1989; Skinner, 1982). Scores range from 0 to 10, with a score of 3 or more being suggestive of a drug problem. As also discussed in Chapter 4, the information on the DAST-10 is used in Session 1 to provide personalized feedback to clients about the seriousness of their drug use prior to treatment (see the last page of Client Handout 4.2).

Drug Use History Questionnaire

If detailed drug use information is needed, the Drug Use History Questionnaire (DUHQ; Appendix C) can reliably provide information about clients' lifetime and recent drug use (years used, route of administration, frequency of use, year last used) (Martin & Wilkinson, 1989; L. C. Sobell, Kwan, & Sobell, 1995; Wilkinson, Leigh, Cordingley, Martin, & Lei, 1987). The DUHQ is other-administered and takes about 3 to 5 minutes. The DUHQ uses a card sort to help clients accurately recall their drug use. The following is an example of how to explain the completion of the DUHQ. Clients' answers are recorded on the form (see Appendix C).

> *"Now we are going to look at your past and present use of different drugs. I have several cards here with the names of different drugs on them which I'd like you to sort into two piles. The first pile would include drugs that you have* **never used,** *not even once, and the second would be drugs you've* **used at least once.** [Client sorts cards into two piles.]
>
> *"Now, I'd like you to take the cards with the names of drugs on them that you said you used at least once and sort these into two more piles—the first is drugs that you* **used just once or on an experimental basis,** *and the second pile would be those drugs that you have used* **more frequently.** [Client sorts into two additional piles.]
>
> *"Now, I want to ask you a few questions about those drugs that you used more frequently."*

Readiness Ruler

The readiness ruler, a motivational interviewing scaling tool, is usually used when first interviewing clients or at the assessment. Because clients come to treatment with different levels of motivation or readiness to change, this simple state measure (i.e., readiness at the present time) allows therapists to assess a client's ambivalence about changing. In the following example, a therapist asks a client to give voice to where he or she is in terms of readiness to change.

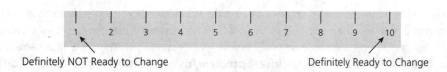

Definitely NOT Ready to Change   Definitely Ready to Change

> *"On a scale from 1 to 10, where 1 is not ready to change and 10 is very ready to change, what number best reflects how ready you are* **at the present time** *to change your* **[insert problem/risky behavior; e.g., alcohol or drug use]***?"*

The readiness ruler can also be used motivationally to ask clients to assess their own progress during therapy (i.e., *"Compared with a month ago, where are you now regarding your readiness to change?"*); to increase their self-efficacy (i.e., *"How did you get from a 4 to a 6? How do you feel about the changes you've made?"*); and to identify the steps necessary for change (i.e., *"What would it take for you to go from a 6 to a 7?"*).

Where Are You Now Scale

The Where Are You Now Scale (Client Handout 3.6) is a motivational scaling tool that asks clients to provide a subjective evaluation of the severity of the problem for which they are seeking treatment. As a state measure, it can be used multiple times over the course of treatment. Therapists can introduce this scale to clients by saying, *"Several times throughout our sessions I am going to ask you to evaluate your alcohol or drug use* [insert problem/risky behavior] *using a 10-point scale, where 1 is the worst ever and 10 is no longer a concern."* In addition to asking clients for a subjective evaluation of their current problems, the form also asks them how they were able to make changes. The following dialogue shows how a therapist could use this scale at the assessment and during treatment.

USING THE WHERE ARE YOU NOW SCALE

ASSESSMENT INTERVIEW

"On a scale from 1 to 10, where 1 is the worst ever and 10 is no longer a concern, how would you rate your [insert problem/risky behavior; e.g., alcohol or drug use] *a year ago and how would you rate it now?"*

At the assessment, some clients will rate their problems as having gotten worse prior to entering treatment (i.e., 5 to a 2). In such cases, the therapist can ask, *"How did you go from a 5 a year ago to a 2 now?"* Such prompts are intended to allow clients to explain how their problem worsened.

Alternatively, some clients will rate their problems as less serious when entering treatment because they have already taken steps to change. In those cases, the therapist can ask, *"How did you go from a 2 a year ago to a 4 now?"* A helpful follow-up question is, *"What would it take to go from a (# they are at now) to a (higher #)?"* The client's answer to the preceding question will often suggest strategies for future progress (e.g., *"If I stop driving by the bar on the way home from work that might work."*).

DURING TREATMENT

After the assessment session, therapists can use the Where Are You Now Scale to have clients compare the number they selected in the previous session with the number they currently selected (e.g., Session 2 vs. assessment, Session 4 vs. Session 2): *"When you first came into treatment, I asked you to rate your* [insert problem/risky behavior; e.g., alcohol or drug use]. *Again, using the same 10-point scale, where 1 is the worst ever and 10 is no longer a concern, how would you rate your* [insert problem risky behavior; e.g., alcohol or drug use] *today?"*

To allow clients to give voice to the change process, therapists can follow up and ask, *"How did you get from a (# given at previous session) to a (# now)?"*

OTHER QUESTIONS FOR CLIENTS WHO HAVE MADE CHANGES

- *"What has changed?"*
- *"How were you able to make the change?"*

- *"How do you feel about the change?"*
- *"What would it take to make additional changes?"*

OTHER QUESTIONS FOR CLIENTS WHO HAVE NOT CHANGED OR CHANGED VERY LITTLE

- *"What obstacles have you encountered in trying to change?"*
- *"What do you think needs to happen in order for you to change?"*
- *"Where will you be in a few years if you do not change?"*
- *"What would be different if you did change?"*

Timeline Followback

The Timeline Followback (TLFB), a psychometrically sound assessment instrument, is the primary assessment and outcome tool used with substance abusers to obtain retrospective estimates of daily alcohol use, illicit drug use, and tobacco use (Agrawal et al., 2008; L. C. Sobell & Sobell, 2003). The TLFB uses a self-report calendar-based format and memory aids to help participants recall their daily use over a specific time period (i.e., number of days) prior to and following treatment. A recent study suggests that for clinical purposes a 3-month pretreatment time window can be used with little or no loss in data accuracy as compared with a 1-year window (Vakili, Sobell, Sobell, Simco, & Agrawal, 2008).The TLFB and related materials are available online (*www.nova.edu/gsc/online_files.html*). Therapist Handouts 3.2 and 3.3 contain the instructions and sample calendars for using the written version of the TLFB for alcohol and drug clients, respectively. As is discussed in Chapter 4, the information collected on the TLFB is used in Session 1 to provide personalized feedback to clients about their alcohol or drug use prior to treatment. For example, feedback can be provided to clients about their alcohol use compared with use by adults in the general population by gender (Client Handout 4.1). Feedback can also be provided on the prevalence of drug use by age for 13 different types of drugs (cigarette use, cocaine and crack use, crack use, hallucinogen use, heroin use, inhalant use, marijuana and hashish use, nonmedical methamphetamine use, nonmedical OxyContin use, nonmedical use of pain relievers, nonmedical sedative use, nonmedical stimulant use, nonmedical tranquilizer use; Client Handout 4.2). Other types of feedback—such as selected health risks, the amount of money spent on alcohol or drugs during a given time period, and the number of calories consumed in alcoholic beverages on a typical day when drinking—can also be generated by the TLFB.

Alcohol Use

The following is a sample dialogue that therapists can have when asking clients to complete the TLFB calendar for their alcohol use.

> *"To help us evaluate your drinking, we need to get an idea of what your alcohol use was like prior to today. To do this, we would like to have you to fill out a calendar showing what your drinking was like over the past* [**insert #**] *days.*

"Filling out the calendar is easy. As you can see in this sample calendar [show the client the sample calendar in Therapist Handout 3.2], *on days when you did drink, you would write in the total number of drinks you consumed. To do this, we want you to record your drinking on the calendar using standard drinks. We use a standard drink format because different alcoholic beverages have different concentrations of alcohol. A standard drink chart is at the top of the calendar. For example, if you had six 12-ounce beers, you would write 6 for that day. If you drank two or more different kinds of alcoholic beverages in a day, such as two beers and three glasses of wine, you would add them up and write a 5.*

"The goal is to get a sense of how frequently you drank, how much you drank, and your patterns of drinking. The idea is to put a number in for each day on the calendar. On days when you did not drink, write a 0.

"While we realize it is not easy to recall things with 100% accuracy, we want you to be as accurate as possible. If you are not sure whether you drank seven or nine drinks on a given day, or whether you drank on a Thursday or a Friday, give us your best estimate. What is important is that seven or nine drinks are very different from two or twenty-five drinks, and seven or nine are different from no drinks. If you have regular patterns to your drinking, such as drinking more on certain days or at certain events, you can use such information to help you recall your drinking. Based on what you report, we will provide you with information about your drinking so that you can use it to make more informed decisions about changing."

Drug Use

When retrospectively evaluating illicit drug use, although reports of the frequency of use have good reliability, reports of the amount used do not have satisfactory reliability. In addition, most clients do not know the actual strength of the illicit drugs they are using. Thus TLFB reports of illicit drug use are limited to frequency of use. The following is a sample dialogue that therapists can have with clients in relation to completing the TLFB calendar for their drug use.

"To help us evaluate your [insert name of the drug] *use, we need to get an idea of what your use was like prior to today. To do this, we would like to have you to fill out a calendar showing what your drug use was like over the past* [insert #] *days. Filling out the calendar is easy. The goal is to get a sense of how frequently you used drugs, and if there are any patterns to your use. The idea is to put a number in for each day on the calendar. As you can see in this sample calendar* [show the client the sample calendar in Therapist Handout 3.3], *on days when you used drugs (except for drugs that are prescribed and used as prescribed) we want you to write a 1, and for days when you did not use drugs write a 0.*

"While we realize it is not easy to recall things with 100% accuracy, we want you to be as accurate as possible. If you have regular patterns to your drug use (e.g., daily or weekend patterns), you can use such information to help you recall your use. Based on what you report, we will provide you with information about your drug use so that you can use it to make more informed decisions about changing."

Brief Situational Confidence Questionnaire

The Brief Situational Confidence Questionnaire (BSCQ) is a psychometrically sound instrument for assessing self-efficacy to resist the urge to use drugs or to drink heavily (Breslin, Sobell, Sobell, & Agrawal, 2000). The BSCQ, which is based on longer versions of the initial questionnaires (Situational Confidence Questionnaire, SCQ-100; Drug Taking Confidence Questionnaire, DTCQ-50) (Annis & Davis, 1988; Sklar, Annis, & Turner, 1997; Solomon & Annis, 1990), assesses clients' confidence or self-efficacy for eight high-risk situations based on Marlatt's relapse taxonomy (Marlatt & Donovan, 2005). For each situation clients rate their confidence in resisting using drugs or drinking heavily on scales ranging from 0% (*not at all confident*) to 100% (*very confident*). Clinically, the BSCQ is used to identify and highlight the clients' three highest risk trigger situations for substance use (i.e., the three situations in which clients are least confident about resisting the urge to drink heavily or use drugs). As discussed in Chapter 4 and Table 4.2, the information from the BSCQ is used to provide personalized feedback to clients in Session 2 (Client Handout 4.7) and Session 4 (Client Handout 4.9). A program that automatically prepares BSCQ graphs based on clients' scores from their ratings entered into the eight high-risk situations is available online (*www.nova.edu/gsc/online_files.html*). At the assessment, the therapist can present the rationale for the BSCQ to clients as follows.

> *"This form asks you how confident you are right now that you could resist the urge to drink heavily or use drugs in eight different types of situations. What we want you to do is to think about each situation and to rate how confident you are at the* **present time** *that you could resist the urge to drink heavily or use drugs in that situation on a scale from 0 to 100, where 0 is not at all confident and 100 is totally confident."*

UTILITY OF HOMEWORK EXERCISES

Starting at the assessment, an important part of the GSC intervention is homework. In fact, homework assignments have been a major element of most cognitive-behavioral interventions for many years. Although research shows a positive relationship between compliance with homework and treatment outcomes (Burns & Spangler, 2000; Kazantzis, 2000), there is variability in how well clients comply with such assignments (Kazantzis & Shinkfield, 2007). Possible factors affecting compliance include what clients perceive as the benefits of completing the homework and their confidence in completing the tasks. Compliance with homework assignments can be increased if therapists explain their rationale and the way the assignment relates to the problem for which clients sought treatment (Dies, 1992).

In our experience, most clients will comply with homework exercises if they understand their rationale. We have found that it is helpful to tell clients that the homework exercises can accelerate their success in changing, as they will be working on changing outside of the sessions. A useful way to start the discussion about homework assignments is to ask clients, *"Why do you think we use homework exercises?"* This can lead to clients giving voice to the reasons that homework is important, and the therapist can then add any reasons not mentioned by clients. The following is a sample dialogue that could be used by therapists in explaining the importance of the homework assignments.

"The homework assignments and self-monitoring logs are intended to help you in several ways. They can help you better understand the treatment approach. They can provide you with feedback about the behaviors you may want to change. They allow you to take an active role in changing and evaluating your progress, and they help you prepare for each session. The reason we ask you to complete homework exercises outside of the sessions is that we have found that this extra effort helps people change."

In the GRIN study (L. C. Sobell et al., 2009) the therapists recorded whether clients completed their homework assignments and self-monitoring logs prior to the sessions. Across all sessions, more than 90% completed both tasks, regardless of whether they were in individual or group therapy. Interestingly, over the four sessions, clients reported that on average they spent almost 6 hours (mean = 5.7) outside of treatment completing their homework exercises and self-monitoring logs. Furthermore, at the end of the four GSC sessions, over 90% of the clients reported that the homework exercises and readings were useful or very useful.

HOMEWORK ASSIGNMENTS GIVEN TO CLIENTS AT THE ASSESSMENT SESSION

Three homework assignments are given to clients at the assessment: (1) self-monitoring logs, (2) decisional balance exercise, and (3) goal evaluations.

Self-Monitoring Logs

The use of self-monitoring logs for alcohol and drug use starts at the assessment and continues throughout treatment. Sample and blank self-monitoring logs and instructions for recording alcohol and drug use are shown in Client Handouts 3.2 and 3.3, respectively. The alcohol self-monitoring logs also contain a standard drink card. Other aspects of alcohol and drug use (e.g., urges to use, situations in which use occurred, thoughts when using) can also be recorded on the logs. The alcohol and drug self-monitoring logs in Client Handouts 3.2 and 3.3, respectively, can be copied and put into a small booklet with a cover. Multiple copies of the blank log page should be included so that clients have a sufficient number of pages on which to record their use over treatment.

Besides collecting information about substance use, self-monitoring serves multiple purposes. It (1) provides an opportunity for clients at the start of each session to talk openly and honestly about their alcohol or drug use since the last session; (2) encourages clients to take responsibility for enacting changes outside of the treatment arena; and (3) provides information that therapists can use to give clients feedback about changes in their alcohol and drug use over the course of treatment (see Chapter 4; Table 4.1, Timeline Followback; and Client Handouts 4.3 and 4.4). The importance of viewing substance use over the course of treatment with clients is that it allows a day of unplanned use to be put in perspective (i.e., a *slight bump in the road* vs. a *downward spiral*). In addition, therapists can use reflective listening to highlight changes that occur, including asking clients how they were able to abstain from or reduce substance use from the time of the last session. The following is a sample dialogue showing how a therapist might introduce the self-monitoring logs at the assessment session.

"This booklet contains self-monitoring logs that we have clients record their alcohol or drug use and urges on during the treatment program. We would like you to fill out the logs every day and bring them with you, as we will go over them at the start of each session. The instructions for the self-monitoring log are on the first page of the booklet. There is also a sample page to show you what a completed log looks like. On days when you did use drugs, write a 1 for that day. If you didn't use drugs on a given day, then write a 0 for that day. In addition, record any urges to use that you experienced, and note places where you did use or where you experienced urges to use. The most important thing is to take some time and complete your self-monitoring logs before each session. The log is easy to fill out and will only take about 5 minutes each day to complete. How does that sound?"

For alcohol and drug clients, a therapist could start the sessions by saying, *"Let's take a look at your self-monitoring logs. How did your week go?"*

Decisional Balance Exercise

The second assignment given to clients at the assessment, which they are asked to complete and bring with them to Session 1, is a decisional balance exercise (Client Handout 3.1). This exercise, which has been used in treatment studies for many years (Center for Substance Abuse Treatment, 1999; Janis & Mann, 1977; Mann, 1972), is a motivational tool that helps clients evaluate in a structured, written manner the pros and cons of changing and of not changing a risky problem behavior. When we give clients a decisional balance exercise, whether it is part of the GSC individual or group treatment, they are told that completing the assignment will help them to get an idea of the *good things* and the *less good things* about their alcohol or drug use and to understand why they might be ambivalent about changing. Looking at all of the pros and cons at the same time can yield a different picture than looking separately at individual costs and benefits.

The decisional balance exercise, which serves as a framework for discussing behavior change and potential obstacles to change, is also useful for treatment planning and goal setting. How the completed decisional balance exercise is used in treatment is discussed in detail in Chapter 4. In explaining the decisional balance homework to clients at the assessment, therapists can present the rationale as follows.

*"This homework assignment is what we call a **decisional balance exercise**, and what I would like you to do is complete it at home and bring it to the next session. It is intended to help you see the whole range of costs and benefits of changing your alcohol/drug use. To do this, we ask you to list the good things and the less good things about changing, as well as the good and less good things about not changing. As you can see, a sample exercise has been completed to give you an idea of how to do this exercise."*

Goal Evaluations

Clients complete goal evaluations on multiple occasions throughout treatment (M. B. Sobell & Sobell, 1986–1987, 1993a, 2005). These goal exercises allow clients to choose their own goal when not contraindicated and to evaluate the importance of their goal and their confidence that they will achieve the goal.

From the standpoint of effective treatment, Miller and Rollnick (2002) discuss why goal choice can be important:

> The fact is that you cannot impose your own goals on a patient. You can offer your best advice, but the patient is always free to accept it or disregard it. Arguing and insisting are more likely to evoke defensiveness than agreement. Again, it makes little sense to work within a motivational interviewing strategy (while first engaging a patient), only to alienate the patient with a rigidly prescriptive style (when negotiating treatment goals). It is far better, we believe, to maintain a strong working alliance with the patient, and to start with the goals toward which he or she is most eager to make progress. If these goals are misguided, it will become apparent soon enough. (p. 120)

Abstinence Goal Evaluation (Client Handout 3.4)

Although we strongly agree with Miller and Rollnick's (2002) statement about the importance of goal choice, we also cannot ignore the fact that there are several situations in which anything other than abstinence is contraindicated for medical, legal, or social reasons. Although research has shown that clients with alcohol problems ultimately select their own goals irrespective of therapists' goal advice (Foy, Nunn, & Rychtarik, 1984; Sanchez-Craig, 1980; Sanchez-Craig et al., 1984; M. B. Sobell & Sobell, 1995), what we advise in cases except where abstinence is contraindicated is to discuss this topic using a motivational interviewing style, which is more likely to reduce resistance.

An abstinence goal evaluation is recommended for the following individuals (Kahan, 1996; M. B. Sobell & Sobell, 1993a): (1) illicit drug abusers; (2) those with legal restrictions on their use of alcohol (e.g., referred from the criminal justice system, on parole); (3) those under the legal drinking age; (4) those who have medical problems that would be exacerbated by alcohol; (5) those on prescription medications for whom alcohol is contraindicated; (6) women who are pregnant, trying to become pregnant, or breast-feeding; and (7) those in a social circumstance in which alcohol use is contraindicated (e.g., drinking might result in a divorce). Clients with contraindications to alcohol or drug use should be advised by their therapists that abstinence is the recommended treatment goal. At the assessment, these clients are given Client Handout 3.4 (Abstinence Goal Evaluation) as homework. This exercise does not ask for a goal specification but rather asks clients to check a box that says that their goal is not to use alcohol or not to use drugs. Furthermore, this evaluation form asks the client to answer two questions assessing his or her motivation regarding the goal: (1) *"At this moment, how important is it for you to achieve your stated goal?"* (0 is *not important at all*, and 100 is *the most important thing in my life I would like to achieve now*); and (2) *"At this moment, how confident are you that you will achieve your stated goal?"* (0 is *I do not think I will achieve my goal*, and 100 is *I think I will definitely achieve my goal*). A way to introduce these goal evaluations is to say, *"The next thing we would like you to complete at home and bring to the next session is a goal evaluation. We would like you to rate the importance of this goal and how confident you are in achieving it."*

Low-Risk Limited Alcohol Use Goal Evaluation (Client Handout 3.5)

Clients with an alcohol problem who have no contraindications to alcohol use (e.g., medical, legal, social, age) are provided with an explicit goal choice (i.e., abstinence or low-risk alcohol use). Such clients are given Client Handout 3.5 and asked to complete it and bring it to Session 1. Clients who select low-risk goals are asked to specify the parameters of their drinking goals on the form (e.g., number of drinking days per week, the amount of drinks per drinking day, specific conditions when drinking will and will not occur). As with an abstinence goal evaluation, the low-risk alcohol use goal evaluation asks clients to rate the importance of their goals and their confidence that they will achieve them. The following is a sample dialogue showing how therapists can introduce the goal evaluation with clients with alcohol problems for whom low-risk drinking is not contraindicated.

> *"The next thing we would like you to complete at home and bring to the next session is a goal evaluation. We want you to select a goal that you think is best for you and realistic. At the next session, I'll be going over your goal with you. In addition, on the second page we would like you to rate the importance of your goal and how confident you are in achieving it. Goals are flexible, so if at some point you decide that this goal isn't working for you, you can change it. The important thing is that you are choosing your goal. If it works, you take the credit for your hard work. If it doesn't work, we can discuss what's getting in the way of your reaching your goal and what the next step is."*

Another example of a goal statement evaluation for alcohol use can be found in the pamphlet *How to Cut Down on Your Drinking* published by the National Institute on Alcohol Abuse and Alcoholism (1996).

With clients for whom low-risk drinking is not contraindicated, the value of having them complete a goal evaluation before discussing goals in Session 2 is that it provides the therapist with knowledge of the client's objectives before the client receives drinking guidelines from the therapist. Although a majority of clients seeking a low-risk drinking goal specify low quantity and frequency limits (i.e., no more than two or three drinks on no more than 3 or 4 days per week) (L. C. Sobell et al., 2009; M. B. Sobell & Sobell, 1993a), some specify amounts that are above the recommended guidelines. Having clients complete the goal evaluation before discussing it in Session 1 reduces the likelihood of clients trying to please their therapists (i.e., having an unrealistic goal).

The approach to goal setting in the GSC treatment model is consistent with evidence-based conclusions we put forth in an editorial in the journal *Addiction* (M. B. Sobell & Sobell, 1995). That editorial was the subject of 11 simultaneously published commentaries by experts in the field. Although a few of the comments were not in favor of giving clients goal choice (e.g., Hore, 1995), none disagreed with the following conclusions:

1. Recoveries of individuals who have been severely dependent on alcohol predominantly involve abstinence.
2. Recoveries of individuals who have not been severely dependent on alcohol predominantly involve reduced drinking.
3. The association of outcome type and dependence severity appears to be independent of advice provided in treatment. (M. B. Sobell & Sobell, 1995, p. 1149)

In other words, the idea that therapists specify clients' treatment goals and that clients then pursue those goals is a *therapist's illusion*. Clients seem to reduce or stop their substance use based on the severity of their problems, rather than on their therapists' advice. Because clients ultimately choose their own goals, we incorporate goal choice into the GSC treatment model where possible (i.e., when not contraindicated). The provision of goal choice is also consistent with Bandura's (1986) social cognitive theory, which asserts that people will be more committed to goals that they set for themselves than to those set for them by others.

ENDING THE ASSESSMENT SESSION: WHAT STOOD OUT?

At the end of each session and prior to scheduling the next session, all clients are asked the following question, *"We have talked about a lot of things today. What one or two things stood out for you?"* This question is used because it allows clients to give voice to what occurred in the session. Our experience has been that clients' responses are often enlightening and sometimes surprising. It is also common to have clients at the assessment session report that what stood out was the motivational interviewing style used by the therapist (e.g., *"I didn't feel judged"* or *"I was listened to"*).

SUMMARY

The GSC treatment model views assessment as the start of treatment, as well as an information-gathering process. Starting at the assessment, therapists use a motivational interviewing style to interact with clients, to collect information, and to express empathy, which in turn leads to developing a working alliance with clients. Emphasis is placed on using assessment instruments that can provide clients with feedback and information with which to make better informed decisions. Sample dialogues illustrating how to present personalized feedback using the assessment measures and questionnaires are presented in the next chapter. Finally, homework assignments given at assessment were also discussed as a way to facilitate treatment and further empower clients to take responsibility for guiding their own change.

Objectives, Materials Needed, Procedures, and Client Handouts
Assessment Session for Group and Individual Therapy

SESSION OBJECTIVES

- Gather background and substance use history information.
- Gather data to be used for feedback in treatment.
- Describe treatment approach.
- Give homework and instructions for Session 1.

ASSESSMENT MEASURES

- Core assessment: Background and problem history information (agency or therapist determined)
- Alcohol Use Disorders Identification Test (AUDIT; Appendix A)
- Drug Abuse Screening Test, 10-item version (DAST-10; Appendix B)
- Timeline Followback (Therapist Handout 3.2 for alcohol use; Therapist Handout 3.3 for drug use)
- Drug Use History Questionnaire (DUHQ; Appendix C) and card sort
- Readiness ruler
- Brief Situational Confidence Questionnaire (BSCQ; Appendix D)
- Where Are You Now Scale form (Client Handout 3.6)
- Decisional balance exercise (Client Handout 3.1)
- Goal evaluation form (abstinence: Client Handout 3.4; low-risk limited drinking: Client Handout 3.5)
- Self-monitoring logs (alcohol use: Client Handout 3.2; drug use: Client Handout 3.3)
- Introduction to groups (Client Handout 5.1 for clients who will participate in group therapy)

OVERVIEW OF ASSESSMENT SESSION

- Introduction, confidentiality, informed consent to treatment.
- Explain key points of treatment approach as shown below (e.g., GSC: Time limited with additional sessions if needed; homework exercises and self-monitoring logs completed outside of sessions; feedback from the assessment measures; learning to use a problem-solving approach to deal with problems; taking responsibility for changing and guiding own change plan).

"The Guided Self-Change program helps you guide your own change and is designed to have you take responsibility for your own change. You will learn how to use a problem-solving approach to deal with your alcohol or drug use and other problems. As part of the program, we are going to ask you to complete some short readings and homework exercises and to keep records of your alcohol and drug use and urges. When people work on things outside of sessions and bring them back in, it helps accelerate their change. For that reason, it is very important to do the assigned homework exercises. The program consists of four semi-structured sessions plus today's assessment. In the fourth session, we'll review your progress and you can decide at that time whether you would like more sessions. One month after your last session I will call you to see how you are doing."

(cont.)

- Purpose of assessment: To gather information on presenting problem(s).
- For clients who will be participating in group therapy, discuss any concerns about being in a therapy group.
- End of assessment interview: Ask what stood out today, ask for questions, schedule next session.

ASSESSMENT PROCEDURES

- Introduction: Start with an open-ended discussion that uses a motivational approach and ask what brought the client to treatment, expectations from treatment, and explain what the assessment session is and how long.
- Explain and get a signed informed consent for treatment.
- Complete core assessment, which includes demographic and substance use history and problems (agency or therapist determined).
- Complete AUDIT, DAST-10, DUHQ, BSCQ, readiness ruler, Where Are You Now Scale.
- Complete 90-day pretreatment Timeline Followback for alcohol or drug use or both.

CLIENT HANDOUTS

- Decisional balance exercise
- Goal evaluation
- Self-monitoring logs

DISCUSS WITH POTENTIAL GROUP THERAPY MEMBERS

- Give introduction to groups handout.
- Discuss group rules, including confidentiality.
- All members need to participate regularly and share information about themselves.
- Members are expected to provide feedback and support to other members.
- Research has found that groups are as effective as individual therapy.

COMPLETE BEFORE SESSION 1

- Prepare personalized feedback on alcohol use (Client Handout 4.2) or drug use (Client Handout 4.3) or, if applicable, both.
- Prepare personalized BSCQ graph for Session 2 (Client Handout 4.7).
- For group clients, make enough copies of Client Handout 5.1 to distribute to all members at the first group meeting.

Timeline Followback Instructions
and Sample Calendar for Alcohol Use

To get an idea of what your alcohol use was like in the last **past** ___ **days**, we would like you to fill out the attached calendar.

TO START

1. Write in **TODAY'S DATE** and **YESTERDAY'S DATE** at the top of the calendar.

2. **Put an X on TODAY'S DATE**, but do **NOT** enter a number of drinks for "today" or any day after today.

3. Starting with **YESTERDAY**, go through the calendar and write the **number of standard drinks** that you drank for **each day** on the calendar. For any day where you drank **no alcohol, write "0."**

4. Below is a **Standard Drink Conversion Chart** that will make it easier for you to record your drinking.

SAMPLE CALENDAR   Write in Today's and Yesterday's Date

ID: 9-999   **Today's Date** June 22, 2010

Start Date: (Day 1) 05/31/10   **End Date: (Yesterday)** June 21, 2010

TIMELINE FOLLOWBACK CALENDAR

1 Standard Drink is Equal to

 One 12 oz. can/bottle of beer   One 5 oz. glass of regular (12%) wine   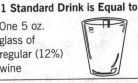 1½ oz. of hard liquor (e.g., rum, vodka, whiskey)   1 mixed or straight drink with 1½ oz. hard liquor

PLEASE READ THE INSTRUCTIONS BEFORE YOU FILL OUT THE CALENDAR

Sun	Mon	Tue	Wed	Thurs	Fri	Sat
30-May	31-May	1-Jun	2-Jun	3-Jun	4-Jun	5-Jun
	Memorial Day 3	1	0	0	3	1
6-Jun	7-Jun	8-Jun	9-Jun	10-Jun	11-Jun	12-Jun
2	0	0	0	0	0	4
13-Jun	14-Jun	15-Jun	16-Jun	17-Jun	18-Jun	19-Jun
0	0	01	0	0	0	1
20-Jun	21-Jun	22-Jun	23-Jun	24-Jun	25-Jun	26-Jun
2	0	X				

Place an X on today, and fill in every day BEFORE today

(cont.)

WHAT TO FILL IN

- When you did drink, you would write in the total number of standard drinks you had on that day.
- When you did not drink, you would write a **"0."**
- **THE IMPORTANT THING IS TO WRITE SOMETHING IN ON EACH DAY, EVEN IF IT IS A "0."**

WE WANT YOU TO RECORD YOUR DRINKING ON THE CALENDAR USING STANDARD DRINKS

For example

- To help you, we want you to use a **Standard Drink conversion**
  1 Standard Drink =
  One 12 oz. beer (5%)
  One 5 oz. glass of wine (11–12%)
  1½ oz. of hard liquor or spirits straight (40%)
  1½ oz. of hard liquor or spirits in a mixed drink (40%)
- If you had six 12-oz. beers, write **6** in for that day.
- If you drank more than one kind of alcoholic beverage in a day, such as two 12-oz. beers and three 5-oz. glasses of wine, you would write **5** in for that day
- **Holidays** are marked on the calendar to help you recall your drinking. You can also think about how much you drank on personal holidays and events such as birthdays, vacations, and parties.

YOUR BEST ESTIMATE

- **Filling out the calendar is not hard!**
- If you are not sure whether you drank three or six drinks or whether you drank on a Thursday or a Friday, give it your best estimate.
- **We recognize people will not have perfect recall, just try to be as accurate as possible.**

Timeline Followback Instructions and Sample Calendar for Drug Use

Primary Drug for Which You Sought Treatment _____

- The following questions relate to the use of the primary drug for which you sought treatment. **When you see the word _drug_**, it means the primary drug for which you sought treatment.
- To get an idea of what your drug use was like in the **past _____ days**, we would like you to fill out the attached calendar.
- The idea is that for **each day** on the calendar we want you to indicate whether you **used** or **did not use** the primary drug for which you sought treatment.

TO START

1. Write in **TODAY'S DATE** and **YESTERDAY'S DATE** at the top of the calendar.
2. **Put an X on TODAY'S DATE**, but do **NOT** enter a number for "today" or any day after today.
3. Starting with **YESTERDAY**, go through the calendar
   a. On days when you **did not use drugs**, write a "**0**" in the box
   b. On days when you **did use drugs**, write a "**✓**" in the box

SAMPLE CALENDAR

ID: 9-999

Start Date: (Day 1) 09/03/10

Write in Today's and Yesterday's Date

Today's Date _October 2, 2010_

End Date: (Yesterday) _October 1, 2010_

SUN	MON	TUES	WED	THURS	FRI	SAT
			1-Sept	2-Sept	3-Sept	4-Sept
					_O_	_O_
5-Sept	6-Sept	7-Sept	8-Sept	9-Sept	10-Sept	11-Sept
_O_	Labor Day ✓	✓	✓	_O_	_O_	✓
12-Sept	13-Sept	14-Sept	15-Sept	16-Sept	17-Sept	18-Sept
✓	✓	_O_	✓	✓	_O_	✓
19-Sept	20-Sept	21-Sept	22-Sept	23-Sept	24-Sept	25-Sept
✓	_O_	_O_	_O_	_O_	✓	✓
26-Sept	27-Sept	28-Sept	29-Sept	30-Sept	1-Oct	2-Oct
_O_	_O_	✓	_O_	_O_	_O_	X

For all days, fill in either a "✓" if you used any drugs on a given day or a "0" if you did not use any drugs

(cont.)

WHAT TO FILL IN

- When you did use the primary drug for which you sought treatment
  - On days when you **did not use drugs**, write a **"0"** in the box
  - On days when you **did use drugs**, you write a **"✓"** in the box
- **THE IMPORTANT THING IS TO WRITE SOMETHING IN ON EACH DAY, EVEN IF IT IS A "0."**
- **Holidays** are marked on the calendar to help you recall your drug use. You can also think about your drug use in relation to personal holidays and events such as birthdays, vacations, and parties.

YOUR BEST ESTIMATE

- **Filling out the calendar is not hard!**
- If you are not sure whether you used drugs on a given day, or whether you used on a Thursday or a Friday, give it your best estimate.
- **We recognize people will not have perfect recall, just try to be as accurate as possible.**

Decisional Balance Exercise

THE BEHAVIOR I AM THINKING OF CHANGING IS:

_____

WEIGHING DECISIONS

When people weigh decisions, they look at the **costs and benefits** of the choices they can make. **Remember that having mixed feelings often occurs when making decisions.**

DECISIONAL BALANCING

Many people change on their own. When they are asked what brought about the change, they often say they just **"thought about it,"** meaning they evaluated the consequences of their current behavior and of changing before making a final decision.

You can do the same thing with the costs of changing on one side and the benefits of changing on the other side. This exercise will help you look at the good things and less good things about changing.

To change, the scale needs to tip so the costs outweigh the benefits.

Weighing the pros and cons of changing happens all the time—for example, when changing jobs or deciding to move or get married.

DECISION TO CHANGE EXERCISE

One thing that helps people when thinking of changing is to list in one place the benefits and costs of changing or continuing their current behavior. Seeing the full array of costs and benefits can make it easier to decide if you should change. Below is an example of a Decision to Change Exercise.

EXAMPLE: DECISION TO CHANGE EXERCISE

	Changing	Not Changing
Benefits of	• Increased control over my life • Support from family and friends • Decreased job problems • Improved health and finances	• More relaxed • More fun at parties • Don't have to think about my problems
Costs of	• Increased stress/anxiety • Feel more depressed • Increased boredom • Sleep problems	• Disapproval from friends/family • Money problems • Damage close relationships • Increased health risks

(cont.)

DECISION TO CHANGE EXERCISE: IT'S YOUR TURN

Fill in the costs and benefits of changing and of not changing. Compare them, and ask yourself **are the costs worth it?**

	Changing	**Not Changing**
Benefits of		
Costs of		

IT'S YOUR DECISION

The next page asks you to list the most important reasons why you want to change. **You are the one who must decide what it will take to tip the scale in favor of changing.**

(cont.)

The most important reasong I want to change is:

_____

_____

_____

_____

_____

_____

_____

If someone gave you $5 million to change the behavior you are thinking about changing for just one day, would you change, and why?

_____

_____

_____

_____

_____

_____

_____

What steps would you have to take to achieve the change and thus receive the $5 million?

_____

_____

_____

_____

_____

_____

_____

Self-Monitoring Logs for Alcohol Use

MONITORING YOUR ALCOHOL USE

SELF-MONITORING is an important part of this program. It can help you

- Record your drinking more accurately because you are writing down what you drink more frequently.
- Evaluate your progress toward your goals. Even when you don't drink, you record a "0" for that day.
- Identify high-risk situations by looking at days on which you drank heavily. Such information allows you and your therapist to develop better coping strategies and alternatives for problem drinking situations.
- Identify situations in which you did not drink or you limited your drinking.

Although self-monitoring might appear time-consuming, keeping records of certain activities is not unusual. Athletes, salespeople, stockbrokers, and others keep track of their progress. **Keeping track of your behavior can help you achieve your goals.**

Although self-monitoring requires some time and commitment, clients who have self-monitored their drinking report that it provides a better understanding of how much they drink and of situations related to their drinking.

- We want you to keep track of your daily drinking and to **bring your records to each session.**
- It is important to keep accurate records. **There are no rights or wrongs** in recording what you drink.
- Self-monitoring is intended to **help you** and **your therapist look at how you are changing.**

INSTRUCTIONS

Remember to bring your completed logs to your next appointment.

At the top of the form, write your name and treatment goal in the spaces provided. If you will also be monitoring drug use other than alcohol, write the name of the drug in the space provided.

For Each Day

- Starting on the day of your assessment, write the **Date** in the first column on the line that corresponds with the day of the week. For example, if you were seen on Wednesday, Nov. 9th, write Nov. 9 on the line that has Wednesday in the first column
- Next, calculate the number of drinks you had that day and include **Beer, Hard Liquor, and Wine.** Then total the number of drinks at the end of each day and write this amount in the **Total No. of Drinks** column. If you don't drink on a day, then write "0" in that day's column. At the end of the week, there is a space at the bottom of the column that says **Total No. of Drinks.** At the end of the week, in that space enter the total number of drinks you had that week.
- If you used a second drug on a day, write **"Y"** for yes in the column **Was a Second Drug Used?** If you didn't use a second drug on a day, write **"N"** for no in that column.
- In the next column, **Did Your Drinking Cause You Problems?,** answer with either **"Y"** for yes or **"N"** for no.

(cont.)

- In the column **Any Urges to Drink?**, answer with either **"Y"** for yes or **"N"** for no.
- In the column **Situations Related to Your Alcohol Use or Urges to Drink?**, check where you were and who you were with when you used alcohol or felt a desire to drink. In the last column, you can note **What Thoughts or Feelings Were You Experiencing?** related to drinking or urges. Use the back of each log sheet to make additional notes related to your drinking.

An example of a completed sheet is on the next page. To increase recording accuracy, it is important to record your drinking for each day rather than trying to recall it at the end of a week.

DRINKING LOG	ONE STANDARD DRINK =
STANDARD DRINK CONVERSIONS **WINE** 1 bottle (25 oz./750 ml) = 5 drinks 1 bottle (40 oz./1.14 L) = 8 drinks 1 bottle fortified (25 oz.) = 8 drinks **HARD LIQUOR** 1 pint (16 oz./480 ml) = 11 drinks 1 fifth (25 oz./750 ml) = 17 drinks 1 quart (40 oz./1.14 L) = 27 drinks	 **12 oz. Beer (5%)** **1½ oz. Hard Liquor (whiskey, gin) (40%; 80 proof)** **5 oz. Regular Wine (12%)** **3 oz. Sweet Wine (20%)**

(cont.)

SAMPLE DAILY ALCOHOL SELF-MONITORING LOG

Name: *John Smith*

Goal: *avg. 2 drinks/day, 2 days/week; limit 3 drinks/day 2x/month*

Year: *2010*

Second Drug Name: *Marijuana*

Date — Write Month and Day	Total # of Drinks — If you did not drink on this day, write "0."	Was a Second Drug Used? Y = Yes N = No	Did Your Drinking Cause You Problems? Y = Yes N = No	Any Urges to Drink? Y = Yes N = No	Situations Related to Your Alcohol Use or Urges to Drink? (check all that apply) — Alone	With Others	Private Place	Public Place	When You Had Urges to Drink or Drank, What Thoughts or Feelings Were You Experiencing?
Mon. Jan 4	0	N	N	N					
Tues. Jan 5	0	N	N	N					
Wed. Jan 6	1	Y	N	N					Bored at home. Had 1 beer. Smoked a joint after dinner.
Thur. Jan 7	0	N	N	Y		X		X	Went out to dinner with girlfriend, wanted to drink but didn't.
Fri. Jan 8	9	N	Y	Y		X	X		At a friend's party, felt like enjoying myself, but overdid it.
Sat. Jan 9	5	Y	N	Y	X		X		Worked on the house all day, had beer in afternoon, wine with dinner.
Sun. Jan 10	12	N	Y	Y		X		X	At football game with friends; spent the evening in the bar.

Weekly Total = 27

Use back for additional notes

(cont.)

DAILY ALCOHOL SELF-MONITORING LOG

Name:

Goal:

Year:

Second Drug Name:

Date — Write Month and Day	Total # of Drinks — If you did not drink on this day, write "0."	Was a Second Drug Used? — Y = Yes — N = No	Did Your Drinking Cause You Problems? — Y = Yes — N = No	Any Urges to Drink? — Y = Yes — N = No	Situations Related to Your Alcohol Use or Urges to Drink? (check all that apply)				When You Had Urges to Drink or Drank, What Thoughts or Feelings Were You Experiencing?
					Alone	With Others	Private Place	Public Place	
Mon.									
Tues.									
Wed.									
Thur.									
Fri.									
Sat.									
Sun.									

Weekly Total =

Use back for additional notes

(cont.)

Instructions: Use this space for any additional notes related to your use of or urges to use alcohol.

_____

_____

_____

_____

_____

_____

_____

_____

_____

_____

_____

_____

_____

_____

_____

_____

_____

_____

_____

_____

_____

_____

_____

_____

_____

_____

Self-Monitoring Logs for Drug Use

MONITORING YOUR DRUG USE

SELF-MONITORING your drug use is an important part of this program. It can help you:

- Record accurate information about your drug use and any changes you make.
- Evaluate your progress toward your goals. Even when you don't use, you record a "0" for that day.
- Identify high-risk situations by looking at days on which you used drugs. Such information allows you and your therapist to develop better coping strategies and alternatives for drug use situations.
- Identify situations in which you did not use drugs.

Although self-monitoring might appear time-consuming, keeping records of certain activities is not unusual. Athletes, salespeople, stockbrokers, and others keep track of their progress. **Keeping track of your behavior can help you achieve your goals.**

Although self-monitoring requires some time and commitment, clients who have self-monitored their drug use report that it provides a better understanding of how much they use and of situations related to their drug use.

- We want you to keep track of your daily drug use and to **bring your logs to each session.**
- It is important to keep accurate records. **There are no rights or wrongs** in recording what you use.
- Self-monitoring is intended to **help you** and **your therapist look at how you are changing.**

INSTRUCTIONS

Remember to bring your completed logs to your next appointment.

- At the top of the form, write your name and the primary drug for which you are seeking treatment. If you will be monitoring a secondary drug (e.g., cocaine), write the name of the drug in the space provided.

For Each Day

- Starting on the day of your assessment, write the **Date** in the first column on the line that corresponds with the day of the week. For example, if you were seen on Wednesday, Nov. 9th, write Nov. 9 on the line that has Wednesday in the first column
- Next, write **"Y"** for Yes or **"N"** for No in the column **Used Drugs?** for your primary and your secondary drugs.
- Then record the total number of standard drinks of alcohol at the end of each day and write this amount in the **Total No. of Drinks** column. If you did not drink on that day, then write "0" in this column. This column is included because it is helpful to see how your drug and alcohol use are related.
- In the column, **Urges to Use Drugs?** answer by writing **"Y"** for Yes or **"N"** for No.
- In the **Situations Related to Your Drug Use or Urges** column, write down where you were and who you were with when you used drugs or felt a desire to use. In the last column, you can note your **thoughts and feelings** at the time. On the back of each log sheet, space is provided to make additional notes related to any of your drug use situations.

An example of a completed self-monitoring sheet is on the next page. To increase recording accuracy, it is important to record your drug use at the end of each day. If you forget, then record your drug use at the beginning of the next day.

(cont.)

SAMPLE DAILY DRUG USE SELF-MONITORING LOG

Name: *John Smith*

Year: *2010*

Primary Drug Used: *Marijuana*

Second Drug Used: *Cocaine*

Date Write Month and Day	Used Drugs? Y = Yes N = No		Total # of Drinks If no drinking, write "0"	Urges to Use Drugs? Y = Yes N = No	Situations Related to Your Drug Use or Urges (alone, social situation)	Thoughts or Feelings Experienced When Using Drugs or Had Urges
	Primary	Secondary				
Mon. Jan 4	N	N	0	N		
Tues. Jan 5	N	N	0	N		
Wed. Jan 6	Y	N	1	N	At home. Had 1 beer. Smoked a joint after dinner.	Bored
Thur. Jan 7	N	N	0	N	Went to dinner with friends, wanted to drink but didn't.	Anxious, but proud later
Fri. Jan 8	Y	Y	5	Y	At a friend's party, felt like enjoying myself, but overdid it.	Wanted to let loose. Thought I would stop earlier.
Sat. Jan 10	Y	Y	2	N	Worked on car; drank beers.	Felt good, not intoxicated.
Sun. Jan 11	Y	N	8	Y	At football game with friends; spent the evening in the bar.	Wanted friends to like me; after drunk didn't care.

(cont.)

DAILY DRUG USE SELF-MONITORING LOG

Name:

Primary Drug Used:

Year:

Second Drug Used:

Date	Used Drugs? Y = Yes N = No		Total # of Drinks	Urges to Use Drugs?	Situations Related to Your Drug Use or Urges (alone, social situation)	Thoughts or Feelings Experienced When Using Drugs or Had Urges
Write Month and Day	Primary	Secondary	If no drinking, write "0"	Y = Yes N = No		
Mon.						
Tues.						
Wed.						
Thur.						
Fri.						
Sat.						
Sun.						

(cont.)

DAILY DRUG USE SELF-MONITORING LOGS: Additional Notes

Instructions: Use this space for any additional notes related to your use of or urges to use drugs.

_____

_____

_____

_____

_____

_____

_____

_____

_____

_____

_____

_____

_____

_____

_____

_____

_____

_____

_____

_____

_____

_____

_____

_____

_____

_____

Abstinence Goal Evaluation for Alcohol or Drugs

Name: _____   Date: _____

IMPORTANCE AND CONFIDENCE OF CHANGING YOUR DRUG OR ALCOHOL USE:
HOW READY ARE YOU?
PART 1

My goal is to not use (check as appropriate): ___**Alcohol** ___**Drugs** (Primary Drug): _____

People usually have several things that they would like to change in their lives. **In terms of not using alcohol or drugs, please answer the following questions.**

At this moment, how important is it that you do not drink alcohol or use drugs? Use the following scale to indicate your importance rating.

0	25	50	75	100
Not important at all	Less important than most of the other things I would like to achieve now	About as important as most of the other things I would like to achieve now	More important than most of the other things I would like to achieve now	The most important thing in my life I would like to achieve now

The importance of my goal is ___%

Now ask yourself the following questions

1. Is my goal important enough that I will work to achieve it even if progress is slow or difficult?

   ____ **Yes** ____ **No**; if no, describe why not: _____

2. Are there any **competing priorities** that could interfere with my achieving my goal?

   ____ **Yes** ____ **No**; if yes, what are they: _____

At this moment, how confident are you that you will not drink alcohol or use drugs?

Use the following scale to indicate your confidence rating.

0	25	50	75	100
I do not think I will achieve my goal	I have a 25% chance of achieving my goal	I have a 50% chance of achieving my goal	I have a 75% chance of achieving my goal	I think I will definitely achieve my goal

I am ___% confident that I will achieve my goal

Now ask yourself the following questions

1. Considering everything, is my confidence rating realistic?

   ____ **Yes** ____ **No**; if no, indicate why: _____

2. Are there any obstacles I might encounter to achieving my goal?

   ____ **No** ____ **Yes**; if yes, what are they? _____

(cont.)

WHERE DOES YOUR GOAL FIT IN AND HOW READY ARE YOU
TO CHANGE YOUR ALCOHOL OR DRUG USE?
PART 2

- Below are four different combinations of importance and confidence goal ratings.
- Look at your ratings and check **which one of the four combinations best describes how ready you are to not drink alcohol or use drugs.**

1. _____ **Low Importance, Low Confidence:** Such individuals usually do not see change as important nor believe they can succeed in making changes if they tried. Such individuals do not appear very ready to change at the present time.

   If you are in this category, ask yourself what it would take to get you to commit to changing.

2. _____ **Low Importance, High Confidence:** Such individuals typically are confident they can change if they thought it were important but are not sure that they want to change at the present time.

   If you are in this category, ask yourself what it would take to tip the scale in favor of your deciding to change.

3. _____ **High Importance, Low Confidence:** Here the problem is not a willingness to change because such individuals are expressing a desire to change. Instead, the problem is that such individuals typically do not have confidence they could succeed if they tried.

   If you are in this category, ask yourself (1) why you feel you cannot change; (2) what is interfering with your confidence to change; and (3) are there things you can do to increase your confidence?

4. _____ **High Importance, High Confidence:** Such individuals not only feel that it is important to change, but also believe they can succeed and appear very ready to change.

   If you are in this category, then it appears you are at a good stage in the change process.

Goal Choice Evaluation for Alcohol Use

Name: _____ Date: _____

GOAL STATEMENT: ALCOHOL USE
PART 1

People usually have several things that they would like to change in their lives. Changing their drinking can be one of those things. What is your current goal? **Please complete either option 1 or 2.**
Remember your goal can change over time.

My current goal is

> **Option 1:** ____ **NOT TO DRINK AT ALL**. If you checked this goal, GO TO PART 2 on the next page now.

OR

> **Option 2:** ____ **TO DRINK ONLY IN CERTAIN WAYS.** If you intend to drink *in certain ways,* you should know that **1 Standard Drink is equal to**
>
> | | |
> |---|---|
> | • 12 oz. of beer (4–5%) | • 5 oz. of *table* wine (11–12%) |
> | • 1½ oz. of liquor or spirits | • 3 oz. of *fortified* wine (20%) |
>
> If your goal is to drink *in certain ways,* please complete the following statements:
> * On the average day when I do drink, I plan to drink no more than ____ standard drinks per day.
> * During an average week, I plan to drink on no more than ____ days.
> * I plan to drink on less than 1 day per week. Check here: ____
> * **I plan to drink ONLY under the following conditions:**
>
> _____
> _____
>
> * **I plan NOT TO DRINK AT ALL under the following conditions:**
>
> _____
> _____
> _____

(cont.)

IMPORTANCE AND CONFIDENCE OF CHANGING YOUR ALCOHOL USE: HOW READY ARE YOU?
PART 2

Please answer the next two questions with regard to the drinking goal you just described on the previous page.

At this moment, how important is it that you achieve your goal? Use the following scale to indicate your importance rating.

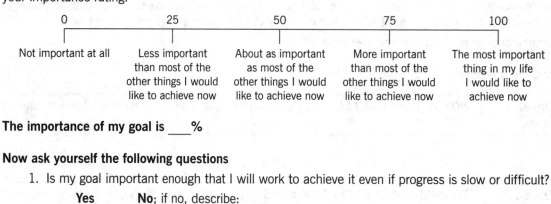

The importance of my goal is ____%

Now ask yourself the following questions

    1. Is my goal important enough that I will work to achieve it even if progress is slow or difficult?

        ___ **Yes** ___ **No**; if no, describe: _____

    2. Are there any **competing priorities** that could interfere with my achieving my goal?

        ___ **Yes** ___ **No**; if yes, what are they? _____

At this moment, how confident are you that you will achieve your goal? Use the following scale to indicate your confidence rating.

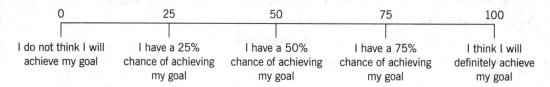

I am ____% confident that I will achieve my goal

Now ask yourself the following questions:

    1. Considering everything, is my confidence rating realistic?

        ___ **Yes** ___ **No**, if no, indicate why: _____

    2. Are there any obstacles to achieving my goal that I might encounter?

        ___ **No** ___ **Yes**; if yes, what are they? _____

(cont.)

WHERE DOES YOUR GOAL FIT IN AND HOW READY ARE YOU
TO CHANGE YOUR ALCOHOL USE?
PART 3

Below are four different combinations of goal importance and confidence ratings.

Look at your ratings and **check which of the four statements best describes how ready you are to change.**

1. _____ **Low Importance, Low Confidence:** Here you are expressing that you are not very confident that you can change and also that it is not very important to you right now.

   If you are in this category, ask yourself what it would take to get you to commit to changing.

2. _____ **Low Importance, High Confidence:** Here you are expressing that you are very confident that you can change, but that it is not that important to you right now.

   If you are in this category, ask yourself what it would take to tip the scale in favor of your deciding to change.

3. _____ **High Importance, Low Confidence:** Here you are expressing that changing is very important, but that do not feel very confident about changing right now.

   If you are in this category, ask yourself: (1) why you feel you cannot change; (2) what is interfering with your confidence to change; and (3) are there things you can do to increase your confidence?

4. _____ **High Importance, High Confidence:** Here you are expressing that you are both very confident that you can change and that it is very important to change right now.

   If you are in this category, it appears you are at a good stage in the change process and are motivated to change.

Where Are You Now Scale

Several times throughout our sessions together I am going to ask you to evaluate your alcohol or drug use using a 10-point scale where **1 = worst ever** and **10 = no longer a concern** (show client the scale):

1	5	10
Worst Ever		No Longer a Concern

1. ASSESSMENT SESSION   Date: _____

On the 10-point scale where 1 = Worst Ever and 10 = No Longer a Concern, how would you rate your alcohol or drug use **a YEAR AGO** and how would you rate it **NOW**?

_____ **RATING A YEAR AGO**

_____ **RATING NOW**

How did you get from (# year ago) to (# Now)? _____

_____

2. SESSION #2   Date: _____

When you first came into treatment I asked you to rate your alcohol or drug use. Using the same 10-point scale where 1 = Worst Ever and 10 = No Longer a Concern, how would you rate your alcohol or drug use **TODAY?**

_____ **SESSION 2 Rating**

How did you get from a (# at assessment) to (# Today)? _____

_____

3. SESSION #4   Date: _____

On two previous occasions, I have asked you to rate your alcohol or drug use. Using the same 10-point scale where 1 = Worst Ever and 10 = No Longer a Concern, how would you rate your alcohol or drug use **TODAY?**

_____ **SESSION 4 Rating**

How did you get from a (# at Session 2) to (# Today)? _____

_____

PART II

Guided Self-Change

A Motivational Cognitive-Behavioral Intervention for Individual and Group Therapy

CHAPTER 4

Guided Self-Change Treatment in an Individual Format

As in our prior reviews, brief interventions again head the list of evidence-based treatment methods, even with brief motivational enhancement approaches removed to a separate category.
—MILLER AND WILBOURNE (2002, p. 275)

This chapter presents a session-by-session description of ways to implement the key elements used in the GSC treatment model with clients seen for individual therapy. At the end of the chapter there are four handouts for therapists (Therapist Handouts 4.1–4.4) that contain an overview of each session's objectives and procedures. Each handout also includes clinical guidelines and dialogues to help therapists conduct the session. Table 4.1 presents a summary of the personalized feedback materials given to clients during Sessions 1–4. The four therapist handouts, 4.1–4.4, were adapted from the GRIN Study protocol (see Sobell & Sobell, 2009).

SESSION 1

Goal Evaluations: Abstinence (Client Handout 3.4) or Goal Choice (Client Handout 3.5)

At the assessment, all clients are given a goal evaluation form (see Chapter 3) to complete and to bring to the first session. Although subsequent sessions begin with a review and discussion of clients' self-monitoring logs, in this session the goal evaluation form is discussed first. Using a motivational interviewing approach, therapists explore clients' answers in an objective, nonjudgmental manner. This is particularly important with clients who do not have severe substance use problems (e.g., problem drinkers, cannabis users who smoke only a few joints on weekends) or who have not been in treatment before. In such cases, just being engaged in an objective discussion about goal choice can minimize or reduce defensiveness.

TABLE 4.1. Personalized Feedback Materials Given to Clients during Sessions 1–4

- *Timeline Followback (TLFB):* The information collected on the Timeline Followback (Agrawal et al., 2008; L. C. Sobell & Sobell, 2003) is used to provide personalized feedback to clients in Session 1 about their alcohol use (*Client Handout 4.1. Personalized Feedback: Where Does Your Alcohol Use Fit In? Individual and Group Session 1*) or drug use prior to treatment (*Client Handout 4.2. Personalized Feedback: Where Does Your Drug Use Fit In? Individual and Group Session 1*). This feedback is used to raise clients' awareness of their alcohol or drug use in relation to national norms. Besides collecting substance use information for each client prior to treatment, data on alcohol and drug use over the course of treatment are collected on the self-monitoring logs (*Client Handouts 3.2 and 3.3*). This information is transferred to a TLFB form, and at the end of treatment a personalized feedback profile is produced of clients' changes from pretreatment to Session 4 in their alcohol use (*Client Handout 4.3. Example of Personalized Alcohol Use Feedback Pretreatment to Session 4: Individual and Group Session 4*) or drug use (*Client Handout 4.4. Example of Personalized Drug Use Feedback Pretreatment to Session 4: Individual and Group Session 4*).

- *Alcohol Use Disorders Identification Test (AUDIT):* Clients' responses to the 10-item version of the AUDIT questionnaire (Gavin et al., 1989; Skinner, 1982) are scored according to the template in Appendix A. In Session 1, based on their answers to the AUDIT, clients with alcohol problems are provided personalized feedback in a motivational interviewing manner that reflects the seriousness of their alcohol problems over the preceding year (*Client Handout 4.1. Personalized Feedback: Where Does Your Alcohol Use Fit In? Individual and Group Session 1*).

- *Drug Abuse Screening Test (DAST-10):* Clients' responses to the 10-item version of the DAST questionnaire (Gavin et al., 1989; Skinner, 1982) are scored using the template in Appendix B. In Session 1, based on their DAST-10 answers, clients with drug problems are provided personalized feedback in a motivational interviewing manner that reflects the seriousness of their drug problems over the preceding year (*Client Handout 4.2. Personalize Feedback: Where Does Your Drug Use Fit In? Individual and Group Session 1*)

- *Brief Situational Confidence Questionnaire (BSCQ):* The BSCQ (Breslin et al., 2000), a state measure of a client's confidence or self-efficacy to resist drinking heavily or using drugs, is used to identify and highlight clients' three highest risk situations (i.e., where they are least confident to resist the urge to drink heavily or use drugs). This chapter contains two examples of the BSCQ feedback given to clients. The first, based on the BSCQ administered at the assessment session, is given to clients in Session 2 (*Client Handout 4.7. Sample BSCQ Alcohol or Drug Use Profile at Assessment: Individual and Group Session 2*). As part of Session 2, this first BSCQ profile is compared with what the clients listed as their two high-risk triggers in the exercise on identifying triggers (*Client Handout 4.6. Individual and Group Session 2*). The three highest risk triggers on the client's BSCQ profile are classified into one of six different BSCQ profiles (see Table 4.2, BSCQ: Eight Categories of High-Risk Situations and Shorthand Names of Profiles). Figure 4.2 contains sample profiles of the six different BSCQ profiles (e.g., good times, testing control). These profile names, intended to capture the three individual high-risk triggers on the BSCQ, also typically reflect the two high-risk situations described in the triggers exercise (M. B. Sobell & Sobell, 1993a). Whereas the BSCQ triggers are generic in nature, the two triggers identified by clients are related to actual situations they have experienced over the previous year. Clients are told that the names of the BSCQ profiles (e.g., *negative affect, good times;* Table 4.2) are intended to provide them with a shorthand label for easier recognition of triggers that they may encounter. At Session 4, clients are provided with feedback based on the BSCQ again. This time the feedback is comparative and uses the client's BSCQ answers at the assessment and Session 3 (*Client Handout 4.9. Sample Comparative BSCQ Alcohol or Drug Use Profiles from the Assessment and Session 3: Individual and Group Session 4*).

- *Readings and Homework Assignments:* The readings and related homework assignments are intended to augment the treatment in terms of saving time, enhancing the continuity of treatment over sessions, and encouraging clients to take responsibility for implementing changes outside of the treatment sessions. The exercises used in the GSC treatment model include:
  - **Homework for Session 1: Exercise 1 Decisional Balance Exercise** (Client Handout 3.1)
  - **Homework for Session 2: Reading on Identifying Triggers** (Client Handout 4.5)
  - **Homework for Session 2: Exercise on Identifying Triggers** (Client Handout 4.6)
  - **Homework for Session 3: Exercise on Developing New Options and Action Plans** (Client Handout 4.8)

Abstinence

Although clients ultimately choose their own goals, therapists are an important source of information and recommendations. For alcohol use, therapists advise clients of any medical, legal, or social contraindications to low-risk limited drinking. Medical contraindications (Kahan, 1996; U.S. Department of Health and Human Services and U.S. Department of Agriculture, 2005) include all health conditions and diseases exacerbated by alcohol consumption (e.g., hepatitis, gout, diabetes, hypertension) and situations in which alcohol consumption can be dangerous (e.g., pregnancy, breast-feeding). Alcohol can also interfere with the metabolism of some prescription drugs by reducing their effectiveness (e.g., antibiotics, antiepileptics) or by enhancing their effects (e.g., benzodiazepines). Other contraindications can be social, such as ultimatums from others (e.g., spouses, family, employers). Legal contraindications include being prohibited from drinking (i.e., a condition of probation or parole) and underage drinking. Readers are referred to Chapter 3 for an in-depth discussion of goal evaluations and contraindications to alcohol use. The topic of low-risk limited drinking is not introduced with clients who have contraindications to drinking because it could undermine their choice of abstinence. It is important that clients view abstinence as a choice because if a slip occurs, then they can choose to stop using.

For legal reasons, clients who use illicit drugs are advised to be abstinent. Therapists also explain to clients with abstinence goals the importance of discussing any alcohol or drug use that occurs during treatment. For honest reporting to occur, it is important for therapists to develop a positive therapeutic relationship with clients. A motivational interviewing approach, which is part of the GSC treatment model, can facilitate this alliance. Substantial evidence demonstrates that when clients are in a clinical setting in which confidentiality is assured and no adverse consequences result from being honest, their self-reports are generally accurate (reviewed in Babor, Steinberg, Anton, & Del Boca, 2000). In other words, when therapists are seen as nonjudgmental and when clients believe that honest reporting will not result in negative consequences, their self-reports can be trusted.

Low-Risk Limited Drinking

Clients with alcohol problems who do not have contraindications to drinking can choose a low-risk limited drinking goal. Over the years, low-risk limited drinking guidelines have varied (Dufour, 1999; International Center for Alcohol Policies, 1998; National Institute on Alcohol Abuse and Alcoholism, 2007). Based on the literature, we have recommended limits of no more than three standard drinks on no more than 4 days per week (M. B. Sobell & Sobell, 1993a). Because women and older adults have a smaller proportion of body water than adult men, some guidelines are gender or age-based (e.g., women and older adults should not consume more than one standard drink per day; men should not consume more than two standard drinks per day; National Institute on Alcohol Abuse and Alcoholism, 1996; U.S. Department of Health and Human Services and U.S. Department of Agriculture, 2005). The guidelines we use, which recommend a limit on both the frequency and quantity of drinking, have the advantage of avoiding daily drinking, which may result in greater tolerance to alcohol than less frequent drinking (Kalant, 1987; Suwaki et al., 2001).

1 STANDARD DRINK *(14 G ABSOLUTE ETHANOL)* =

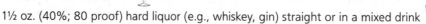

12 oz. (5%) beer

5 oz. (12%) regular wine

1½ oz. (40%; 80 proof) hard liquor (e.g., whiskey, gin) straight or in a mixed drink

Part of the goal evaluation includes a discussion with clients about the reasons they seek to engage in low-risk limited drinking. In this regard, the main reasons for drinking should be social rather than drinking for the effects (i.e., to become intoxicated). If clients are drinking for the effects, over time tolerance is likely to result in their exceeding their limits and increasing their drinking to achieve the desired effects (Maisto, Henry, Sobell, & Sobell, 1978). Consequently, drinking to feel intoxicated is considered high risk. Finally, as part of their goal evaluation, clients are also asked to specify situations that are high and low risk for drinking.

Goal Importance and Confidence

The goal evaluation form also asks clients to rate the importance of and their confidence (i.e., self-efficacy) in achieving their goal. It is common to have clients indicate that meeting their goals is not the most important thing in their lives (i.e., other things, such as their health, have a higher priority). Moreover, for persons whose problems are not severe, achieving their goals will often compete with other activities in their lives (e.g., relationships, jobs). Asking clients to rate the importance of and their confidence in meeting their goals allows for a discussion of motivating factors and of possible obstacles to change. Low confidence ratings can reflect a lack of perceived skills or problem-solving deficits. After finding out how confident clients are about achieving their goals, the following question can be asked, *"What would have to happen for your confidence to increase from 50% to 60%?"* Clients' answers to such questions often identify potential solutions (e.g., *"If I weren't around my friends who are always using, then my confidence would increase"*). Finally, clients are told that the goal statement will be readministered later in treatment and that they are free to modify or change their goals at any time.

Harm Reduction

Although the vast majority of clients seek realistic goals that fit their circumstances, there will be some who, despite recognizing contraindications to drinking, nevertheless seek to reduce rather than stop. Also, some clients with primary drug problems, especially those using cannabis, will not be willing to commit to abstinence. In such cases, we recommend taking a harm-reduction approach (Berridge, 1999; Erickson, 2007; Lieber, Weiss, Groszmann, Paronetto, & Schenker, 2003; Witkiewitz & Marlatt, 2006). Using this approach, clients are informed at each session that the therapist's advice is to not drink or use drugs. However, they are told that if they decide not to follow this advice, it is extremely important that they report their alcohol or drug use honestly during treatment. Finally, it is important to document in a client's clinical or medical record that he or she was advised to abstain and the reasons on which that recommendation was based. Such an approach, although not ideal, is preferable to clients' not reporting using (thus undermining the trust aspect of the therapeutic relationship), or leaving treatment because the therapist was not willing to consider a harm-reduction goal.

Discussion of Clients' Self-Monitoring Logs (Alcohol: Client Handout 3.2; Drug: Client Handout 3.3)

A natural progression after the goal discussion at the start of Session 1 is to ask clients to discuss how their week went by discussing their self-monitoring logs. The therapist can ask, *"How does your alcohol or drug use over the last week relate to your goal?"* If the fit is poor (e.g., abstinence goal, but drinking or drug use occurred), this lends itself to a discussion of the consistency of the client's goal and behavior (i.e., either behavior or goal needs to change). Unless relevant, a detailed, day-by-day description of the client's drinking or drug use should be avoided. Instead the therapist can say, *"Give me a general picture of what your drinking or drug use was like this past week."*

Personalized Feedback Summaries of Pretreatment Alcohol and Drug Use (Alcohol: Client Handout 4.1; Drug: Client Handout 4.2)

After the goal and self-monitoring log discussion, clients are given a copy of their personalized feedback handouts (i.e., Where Does Your Alcohol/Drug Use Fit In?). Two sample dialogues showing how to discuss the feedback with clients appear next.

EXAMPLE OF PROVIDING FEEDBACK BASED ON CLIENTS' REPORTED ALCOHOL OR DRUG USE FROM THEIR TIMELINE CALENDAR

"As I mentioned last week, at this session we will be providing you feedback about your alcohol and drug use based on the information you provided at the assessment. The first type of feedback is based on your daily alcohol or drug use" [Client Handout 4.1, Where Does Your Alcohol Use Fit In?; Client Handout 4.2, Where Does Your Drug Use Fit In?].

For Alcohol Clients: *We calculated the average number of drinks you reported consuming per week over the past 90 days. Looking at this graph, what does it say about where your drinking fits in compared to U.S. drinking norms for [**insert men or women here**]? What stands out for you?"*

Over the years, we have heard many clients who, after comparing their drinking to national norms, say something like the following:

Client: *"How can my drinking be in one of highest groups? Most of my friends drink as much or more than I do?"*

Therapist: *"It sounds like you are surprised about where your drinking fits in because it is similar to that of your friends. What do you think that says?"*

When therapists ask this question, it has prompted many clients to say that their friends are also heavy drinkers. Considering that most clients' goals will be to not drink or to drink less, the therapist might say, *"What kind of social pressure is there to drink when you are with your friends?"*

For Drug Clients (e.g., cocaine): *"This chart shows you what percentage of people have used cocaine in the past month, past year, and lifetime. Where does your drug use fit in? What stands out for you?"*

When drug clients have been given this kind of feedback about their cocaine use prior to entering treatment, a common response has been *"Wow, most of my friends use cocaine, but these graphs say that only a small percent of people used cocaine last year."* When we hear this, we recommend having the therapist normalize the client's response by saying, *"Your response isn't uncommon. People who use drugs often associate with others who use drugs and thus can easily get the sense that many more people use drugs than actually do."*

Besides the general feedback (e.g., % drinking heavily or using cocaine), the therapist may be aware of other information that can be used in a motivationally enhancing manner to help clients increase their commitment to change (e.g., a medical problem that will be exacerbated by drinking).

The following is another example of how to present feedback based on the assessment information. In this case, the feedback relates to alcohol or drug problem severity scores.

EXAMPLE OF PROVIDING FEEDBACK BASED ON CLIENTS' AUDIT AND DAST-10 SCORES

"If you remember, we asked you many questions about your alcohol and drug use at the assessment, and one thing we had you do was report consequences you experienced related to your alcohol or drug use over the past year. We have taken this information and prepared a personalized feedback summary for you so you can better evaluate your alcohol or drug use. Based on what you reported, we calculated scores that reflect the severity of your alcohol use [AUDIT] or drug use [DAST-10]. What stands out about this graph?" [This feedback is on the last page of Client Handout 4.1 for the AUDIT and Client Handout 4.2 for the DAST-10.]

Some clients who see the AUDIT and DAST-10 feedback graphs will say, *"How can that be?"* For those clients, the therapist could say, *"Let's take a look at what you wrote on the forms."* In this way, the therapist uses the clients' answers to address their surprise. Further discussion can occur from asking the clients to elaborate on their answers to specific questions (e.g., *"Have you or someone else been injured as a result of your drinking?"*; *"Have you neglected your family because of your use of drugs?"*).

A motivational interviewing technique that often works well before providing feedback to clients is *asking permission* (see Chapter 2 for a further discussion about this technique). By asking permission, therapists demonstrate respect for clients. When clients are asked for permission to talk about topics, our experience has been that almost all respond affirmatively. For example, we have seen many clients with alcohol problems who also have hypertension and are not aware that alcohol increases their blood pressure. Rather than lecturing them, the therapist can say, *"I wonder what you know about how alcohol can affect a person's blood pressure?"* Typically, clients either do not know or will say something like, *"Well, it's not good for me."* The therapist can then say, *"Would you be interested in learning more about how drinking can affect people's blood pressure?"* At this time, therapists can hand out relevant pamphlets on the topic at hand. A few clients will not want feedback, and in such cases, therapists can use a motivational interviewing technique called *rolling with resistance* and say, *"Okay, we can talk about this at another time if you like."*

Decisional Balance Exercise: Discussion of the Good and Less Good Things about Changing Alcohol or Drug Use (Client Handout 3.1)

The therapist and client together review the decisional balance exercise that the client completed between the assessment and Session 1. If clients fail to bring in the exercise, we usually have them complete it during the session. The decisional balance exercise provides an excellent opportunity to use motivational interviewing techniques. When discussing clients' responses to their decisional balance exercise, it is important to have clients first discuss the *good things* about their substance use, after which they are asked to discuss the *less good things*. The reason for ordering the discussion in this way is that, as mentioned earlier, many substance abusers come to treatment expecting to be lectured about their behavior and told that they must change, without any recognition by the therapist of why it might be difficult to change.

Starting the decisional balance exercise discussion with an explicit acknowledgement of the positive side of the behavior (e.g., *"What are the good things about your alcohol or drug use?"*) not only highlights ambivalence about change but also makes it acceptable for clients to openly discuss what they get out of their alcohol or drug use (i.e., rewards). Discussing ambivalence can be helpful in building a therapeutic relationship as it allows clients to discuss the attraction (i.e., good things) of the behavior without being judged. In addition, there are reasons to think that having clients write down the costs and benefits of changing and of not changing may make the relationships between the behavior and its negative consequences more salient (Baumeister, 1994). The following example demonstrates how a discussion of a decisional balance exercise can be used to summarize a client's ambivalence and to recognize that making decisions to change can be difficult.

> *"On the one hand, what I hear you saying is that if you don't stop using cocaine with your friends you could end up losing your wife and your children, but on the other hand you have concerns about breaking off relationships with friends you've known for many years. That must make quitting more difficult."*

The Five-Million-Dollar Question

The five-million-dollar question, which is in the second part of the decisional balance exercise, involves asking clients if they would stop using alcohol or drugs (or change any behavior) for one day if they were offered five million dollars. Our experience when asking this question is that almost all clients will say *Yes*, after which the therapist says, *"What does that tell you?"* The usual response is something like, *"I could change if the price were right."* The important point is for clients to recognize that what they have said is that changing is a choice. This can be followed by the therapist asking, *"What would it take for you to tip the scale in favor of changing?"*

In the few cases in which a client says, *"I will not change for any amount of money,"* therapists can say, *"Okay, if you would not change your [insert behavior] for just one day for five million dollars, what one thing would it take for you to change for just one day?"* If the client comes up with a response (e.g., *"If my family were to leave me"*), the therapist can then follow up as in the preceding paragraph, getting the client to say that changing is a choice. If the discussion identifies that the client feels that change will be very difficult, that fact can be acknowledged and normalized by saying, "*A lot of people find changing to be difficult. If it were easy, you wouldn't be here.*"

End of Session: Wrap-Up and What Stood Out

In ending the first session, the therapist gives clients the next homework assignment, which involves conducting a functional analysis of their substance use by describing two high-risk situations (M. B. Sobell & Sobell, 1993a; M. B. Sobell et al., 1976). There are two parts to this homework: the Identifying Triggers reading (Client Handout 4.5) and the Identifying Triggers exercise (Client Handout 4.6). The reading introduces the concept of taking a realistic perspective on change using a diagram of a mountain that shows a person walking up a path to the top (i.e., Mt. Change; see diagram in Session 2). For the two high-risk situations in this exercise, clients are asked to identify setting events (i.e., triggers that set the stage for the behavior to occur) and short-term and long-term consequences. Finally, before scheduling the next session, clients are asked, "*We have talked about a lot of things today. What one thing stood out?*"

SESSION 2

Discussion of Clients' Self-Monitoring Logs (Alcohol: Client Handout 3.2; Drug: Client Handout 3.3)

Unless there is an overriding reason (e.g., client in crisis) to start on another topic, the remaining sessions begin with the therapist asking the client how his or her week went and looking at his or her self-monitoring log. The clients are asked to describe major events during the week and how these affected their substance use or urges to use. Again, it is important not to get bogged down with the details of each day, but rather to discuss notable events. In this regard, the therapist can ask the client to summarize the major events of the past week as related to his or her alcohol or drug use or ask questions related to specifics in the self-monitoring logs (e.g., "*I noticed that last Thursday you felt an urge to drink or use drugs, but you didn't use. How were you able to do that?*").

Discussion of the Identifying Triggers Reading (Client Handout 4.5) and Exercise (Client Handout 4.6)

The Identifying Triggers reading is a brief handout that (1) explains how to complete the Identifying Triggers homework and the related homework for the next session, Developing New Options and Action Plans; and (2) presents a cognitive relapse-prevention perspective on changing (i.e., there may be unplanned substance use during treatment, and how one responds to slips is very important). The reading communicates that changing one's alcohol or drug use often is associated with some ups and downs (Hunt, Barnett, & Branch, 1971; Marlatt & Donovan, 2005; Witkiewitz & Marlatt, 2004). In this regard, it is important for clients to have a realistic perspective on change (i.e., Mt. Change) and to use slips as learning experiences should they occur.

Clients are first asked what stood out about this reading and exercise, as well as the relapse-prevention part of the reading. They are then asked to talk about the two high-risk trigger situations they identified for their alcohol or drug use, including describing the short- and long-term consequences related to those two situations.

What follows is an in-depth discussion of the relapse-prevention aspects of the reading.

Mt. Change and Relapse Prevention

The purpose of the illustration and discussion of Mt. Change in the reading is to provide clients with a realistic perspective on change and to help clients learn that if a slip occurs not to view it as a major setback. Although relapse prevention traditionally has included identification of high-risk situations and skills training for handling risk situations (Marlatt & Donovan, 2005), brief treatments such as GSC do not usually include skills training (although the flexibility inherent in this approach would allow for such training if needed). Familiarizing clients with the cognitive components of relapse prevention is important because substance use problems can be recurrent (see Figure 4.1).

The therapist's discussion of the reading with clients, as is the case for all GSC readings and exercises, is done using a motivational interviewing approach rather than lecturing about the possibility of setbacks. For example, the therapist can say, *"In your homework, there was a diagram called Mt. Change. Why do you think we included it?"* In discussing the possibility of relapse, we have found it useful to start out by likening it to a fire drill. We ask clients, *"Why do you think most schools routinely have fire drills?"* Most clients respond by saying, *"People need*

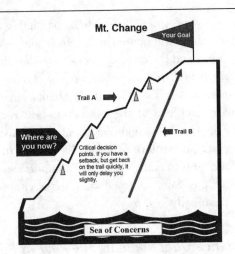

- View recovery as a long-term process (i.e., emphasis is on maintaining motivation if a slip occurs).
- Recognize that slips may occur after treatment and that how individuals deal with them is important to their long-term recovery.
- If slips occur, interrupt them early to minimize consequences and risks.
- If slips occur, use them as learning experiences to prevent similar occurrences in the future (i.e., you have information to identify future high-risk situations and develop alternative coping strategies).
- Construe slips as unfortunate and isolated events rather than as personal failures.
- Learn from the slip and move on (i.e., do not ruminate about slips).

FIGURE 4.1. Cognitive components of the relapse prevention model.

to be prepared should a fire occur." Hearing this, therapists can say, *"That is what this reading is about; although we do not expect problems to occur, it makes sense to think about what to do should a slip occur."*

Learning to Ride a Bike

The process of recovery can be likened to that of learning to ride a bicycle. Using this analogy, clients can be asked if they ever learned how to ride a bike. Because most say *Yes,* the therapist then asks if they ever fell off and what happened (e.g., bruised knee, but they then got back on again). The point for therapists to make here is that changing one's substance use is sometimes like learning how to ride a bicycle. It is a skill. Although some people pick it up right away, others may fall off a few times, but they get back on, and over time they learn how to ride successfully without falling.

Identifying Triggers

Related to the Identifying Triggers reading is the Identifying Triggers exercise (see Client Handout 4.6) that asks clients to identify personal high-risk situations for alcohol or drug use and to evaluate the short- and long-term consequences of using in those situations. What clients are being asked to do in this exercise is to formulate a functional analysis of their alcohol or drug use. They do this by identifying their high-risk situations for drinking or drug use and the associated consequences.

Clients demonstrate a range of competencies when completing this assignment. We begin by asking them what stood out about the homework exercise and ask them to discuss their two high-risk substance use situations and the consequences they identified (e.g., *"Tell me about the trigger situations you described and their consequences"*). Having the homework completed before the session makes treatment more efficient, as clients have already spent some time thinking about their alcohol or drug use. If clients' exercise answers are not very descriptive, they can be expanded on during the discussion. For clients who have difficulty identifying triggers or consequences, therapists can explore this exercise further in the session. An important objective of the exercise is for clients to come away with an understanding of why they use alcohol or drugs in high-risk situations. Such an understanding is vital to developing plans to stop using alcohol or drugs problematically.

Brief Situational Confidence Questionnaire: Review of Personalized High-Risk Profiles for Alcohol or Drug Use (Client Handout 4.7)

In addition to reviewing the two trigger situations identified in the clients' homework, the therapist provides clients with additional feedback about high-risk situations from the BSCQ (Appendix D) that they completed at the assessment. The BSCQ asks clients to rate their confidence (i.e., self-efficacy) on a scale from 0% to 100% that *at the present time* (i.e., state measure) they would be able to resist the urge to drink heavily or use drugs in eight situations often reported as precipitating relapse: *unpleasant emotions, physical discomfort, testing control, urges and temptations, pleasant times with others, conflict with others, pleasant emotions, and social pressure to drink* (Annis, 1986; Marlatt & Gordon, 1985). We have found that the cluster of situations that a client describes as high risk can be given a shorthand label that helps clients to better recall the kinds of situations that tend to be problematic for them.

Table 4.2 lists the eight BSCQ categories of high-risk situations as well as the shorthand BSCQ profile names and descriptions. Figure 4.2 presents sample graphs of each of the six BSCQ profiles. For clients with alcohol problems, research has shown that those who demonstrate positive affect profiles typically have less severe substance use histories, whereas those with more severe histories are more likely to be characterized by negative affect profiles (Cunningham, Sobell, Sobell, Gavin, & Annis, 1995). A sample of a BSCQ profile completed at the assessment and given to clients during Session 2, and a sample of a comparative profile (i.e., changes from assessment to Session 3) given to clients at Session 4 are shown in Client Handouts 4.7 and 4.9, respectively. To create BSCQ profiles similar to the Client Handouts 4.7 and 4.9, readers can use an Excel spreadsheet, which can be downloaded for free at *www.nova.edu/gsc/online_files.html*.

TABLE 4.2. BSCQ: Eight Categories of High-Risk Situations[a] and Shorthand Names of Profiles

High-risk situations

1. Unpleasant Emotions (e.g., *"If I were depressed in general"; "If everything was going badly for me."*).
2. Physical Discomfort (e.g., *"If I would have trouble sleeping"; "If I felt jumpy and physically tense."*)
3. Pleasant Emotions (e.g., *"If something good happened and I felt like celebrating"; "If things were going well."*)
4. Testing Personal Control (i.e., over substance use; e.g., *"If I would start to believe that alcohol or drug use was no longer a problem for me"; "If I would feel confident that I could handle a few drinks or use drugs."*)
5. Urges and Temptations (e.g., *"If I would suddenly have an urge to drink or use drugs"; "If I would be in a situation in which I was in the habit of having a drink or using drugs."*).
6. Conflict with Others (e.g., *"If I had an argument with a friend"; "If I wasn't getting along with others at work."*).
7. Social Pressure to Drink (e.g., *"If someone would pressure me to 'be a good sport' and have a drink"; "If I would be invited to someone's home and they would offer me a drink."*)
8. Pleasant Times with Others (e.g., *"If I wanted to celebrate with a friend"; "If I would be enjoying myself at a party and wanted to feel even better."*)

Shorthand names of profiles

- Good Times: Use is primarily related to positive affective states; for this profile the following two high-risk categories reflect low self-confidence—*pleasant emotions* and *pleasant times with others*.
- Good Times, Social Pressure: Use is primarily related to positive affective states and social pressure; for this profile the *social pressure* category reflects low self-confidence and at least one of the following two high-risk categories also reflect low self-confidence—*pleasant emotions* and *pleasant times with others*.
- Negative Affective: Use is primarily related to negative affective states; for this profile two of the three following high-risk categories reflect low self-confidence—*unpleasant emotions, conflict with others, physical discomfort*.
- Testing Personal Control: Use primarily reflects trying to limit one's alcohol or drug use; for this profile the category of *testing personal control* reflects low self-confidence.
- Affective: Use is primarily related to at least one positive and one negative affective state; for this profile at least one of following three high-risk categories reflects low self-confidence—*unpleasant emotions, conflict with others, physical discomfort*; and at least one of the following two high-risk categories reflects low self-confidence—*pleasant emotions* and *pleasant times with others*.
- Undifferentiated Flat: Use is primarily associated with daily alcohol or drug use; although the self-confidence level can vary, this profile lacks distinct peaks for any of the eight high-risk categories.

[a]Situations clients reported as precipitants to relapse (Marlatt & Donovan, 2005).

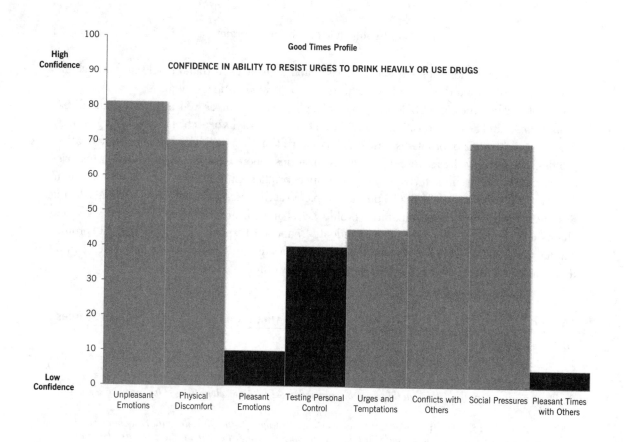

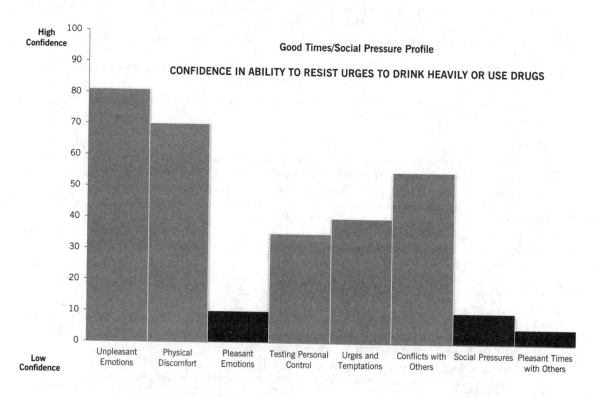

FIGURE 4.2. Sample graphs of the six BSCQ profiles.

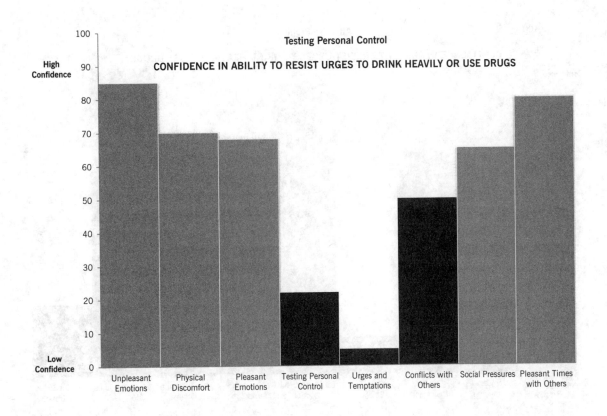

Testing Personal Control

CONFIDENCE IN ABILITY TO RESIST URGES TO DRINK HEAVILY OR USE DRUGS

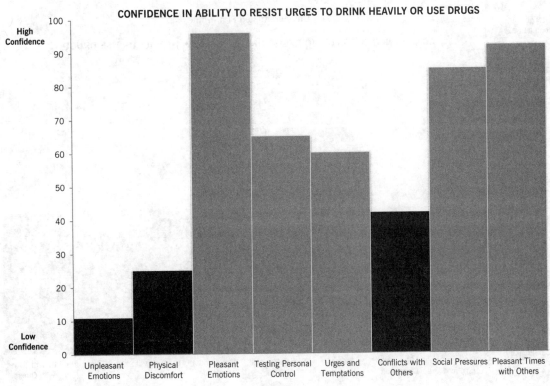

Negative Affective Profile

CONFIDENCE IN ABILITY TO RESIST URGES TO DRINK HEAVILY OR USE DRUGS

FIGURE 4.2. *(cont.)*

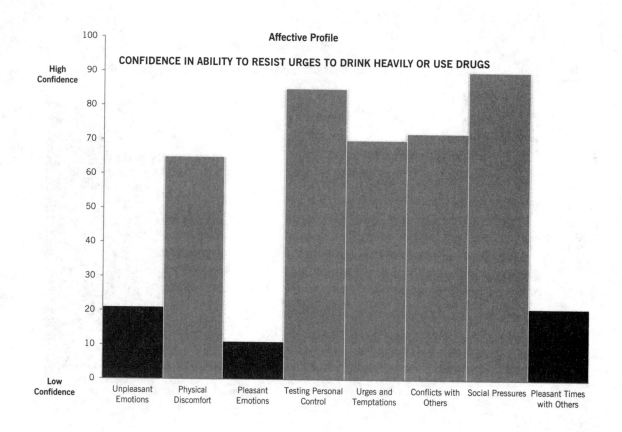

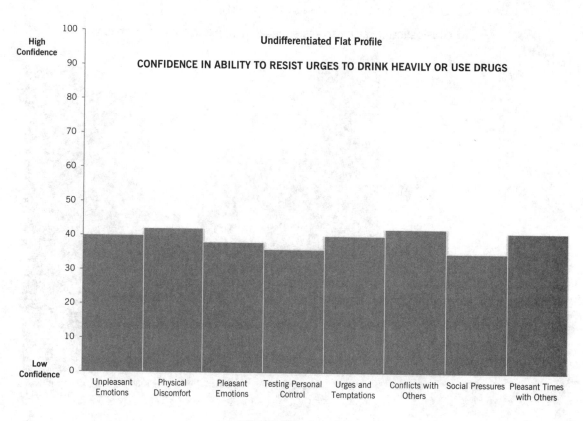

FIGURE 4.2. *(cont.)*

94

An example of how to provide BSCQ feedback to clients follows. This discussion focuses on having clients relate their BSCQ scores and profile (e.g., Good Times/Social Pressure) to the two trigger situations they described in their homework (Client Handout 4.6). Our experience has been that in most cases the trigger situations described in the homework will correspond well with the situations identified as having the lowest confidence on the BSCQ. One time when this does not occur is when all or almost all of the eight situations reflect low confidence (i.e., Undifferentiated). Such profiles often reflect daily heavy alcohol use or daily drug use that by its chronic nature tends not to be situation-specific.

EXAMPLE OF PROVIDING CLIENTS WITH FEEDBACK FROM THEIR BSCQ AT SESSION 2

Note: Prior to this discussion, the therapist completes a BSCQ profile similar to that shown in Client Handout 4.7 containing the client's answers from the assessment interview.

"At the assessment you completed a questionnaire called the Brief Situational Confidence Questionnaire that asked you to rate how confident you were that you could resist the urge to drink heavily or use drugs in eight situations. What I've done is graphed your answers to show you how confident you said you are that you could resist the urge to drink heavily or use drugs in those situations. I also highlighted the three situations in which you indicated you had the least confidence. Looking at your graph, what stands out in terms of high-risk situations related to your alcohol or drug use?

"For those situations that you identified on the scale as high risk, we have found it is easier for people to remember them if we use a summary name. In looking at this graph, what do you see? [Client answers.] *The summary name usually used for a profile like yours is* [**insert shorthand profile name**]."

The following questions can be asked of clients: *"How do the high-risk situations on the graph relate to the two situations you identified in your triggers homework?"* and *"What does this suggest to you?"*

Note: For whatever clients say (e.g., *"I should be more on guard when I am in a situation that involves feeling bad"*), therapists should ask clients the following question:

"What kinds of [**insert the name of the BSCQ profile here; e.g., negative affect**] *situations can you think of that you might encounter over the next few weeks and how might you handle them?"*

Where Are You Now Scale Readministered (Client Handout 3.6)

At the end of this session, we ask clients to again complete the Where Are You Now Scale (Client Handout 3.6) and to compare their current ratings with those they reported at the assessment. This form allows therapists to record clients' repeated ratings using the 10-point scale. Clients' ratings can be used to reinforce progress (e.g., *"How did you get from a 4 at the assessment to a 6 now?"*) and to identify what is needed for further change (e.g., *"What would it take for you to go a step further to a 7 or 8 in the next few weeks?"*).

Homework Assignment: Developing New Options and Action Plans Exercise (Client Handout 4.8)

Before completing Session 2, clients are given another homework exercise (Client Handout 4.8), Developing New Options and Action Plans, to complete and bring to Session 3. This exercise is related to the Identifying Triggers reading and exercise. Taken together, the reading and the two exercises provide instruction in a basic problem-solving approach (D'Zurilla & Goldfried, 1971) to substance use that has always been part of the GSC treatment model (M. B. Sobell & Sobell, 1973, 1993a).

End of Session: Wrap-Up and What Stood Out

Before scheduling the next session, clients are asked, *"What stood out about today's session?"*

SESSION 3

The next two sessions use many of the procedures, questionnaires, and exercises that have been already been discussed at length. Rather than repeating this information, readers can consult the previous material if clarifications are needed. At the beginning of Session 3, clients are asked to complete a second BSCQ and are told that at the next session they will receive feedback comparing their BSCQ answers at the assessment with those in this session.

Discussion of Clients' Self-Monitoring Logs (Alcohol: Client Handout 3.2; Drug: Client Handout 3.3)

After the BSCQ is completed, the session continues with a review and discussion of the client's substance use (or nonuse) between sessions using the self-monitoring logs. As in the previous session, clients are asked to describe major events since the last session and how these affected their substance use or urges to use. Again, it is important not to get bogged down with the details of each day but rather to discuss notable events.

Developing New Options and Action Plans: Discussing Answers to the Homework Exercise for Dealing with High-Risk Trigger Situations (Client Handout 4.8)

The Developing New Options and Action Plans exercise asks clients to address the two trigger situations from their previous homework exercise (Client Handout 4.6) by: (1) identifying options (i.e., strategies, alternative ways of handling the situation) that they could use to deal with such situations other than using substances; (2) evaluating the consequences of using those options; and (3) developing action plans for implementing their chosen options. Whenever possible, it is important to break action plans into small steps, as this allows clients opportunities to recognize progress and therapists opportunities to reinforce clients' progress. Consistent with the GSC treatment's emphasis on empowering clients to take an active role in their treatment, completing the homework constitutes clients' developing their own treatment plan. Most clients will do a good job of developing treatment strategies and plans, but for those who do not, the therapist can help them during the session to develop realistic change plans.

Using a motivational interviewing approach, therapists ask clients to give voice to the change plans described in this homework exercise (e.g., *"Tell me about the options you came up with for resisting social pressure"*). Although the proposed plans are discussed in detail, we also emphasize to clients that the same problem-solving strategy can be used to deal with unanticipated high-risk situations not described in their homework. In other words, clients are made aware that what they are learning is a problem-solving strategy, an approach that can be generalized to future high-risk situations.

Homework Assignments: Putting Options into Practice, Goal Evaluation Revisited, and Request for Additional Sessions

At the end of the discussion of the Developing New Options and Action Plans homework, clients are asked whether there are any high-risk situations that they can think of that might occur between this and the next session. If any situations are identified, clients are asked to formulate plans for dealing with them. Clients are also given another goal evaluation form (Abstinence: Client Handout 3.4; Low-Risk Limited Drinking: Client Handout 3.5) to complete and bring to the next session. As discussed previously, only alcohol clients with no contraindications for drinking are given the goal evaluation form presenting them with a low-risk limited drinking option (Client Handout 3.5).

Finally, although the majority of brief treatments for substance use disorders demonstrate positive treatment outcomes and a substantial proportion of clients demonstrate an early and maintained improvement (Breslin, Sobell, Sobell, Buchan, & Cunningham, 1997), not all clients will improve sufficiently in the short term. Consequently, it is important to be sensitive to individual differences among clients, and thus the length of treatment should be individually tailored. For this reason, the GSC treatment model allows clients to request additional sessions. Rather than approaching the possibility of additional sessions in a discussion in which clients may feel awkward, caught unprepared, or rushed to make a decision, we have found it helpful to give them a Request for Additional Sessions form (Client Handout 4.10) to complete and bring to the next session.

End of Session: Wrap-Up and What Stood Out

Before scheduling the next session, clients are asked, *"What stood out about today's session?"*

SESSION 4

Discussion of Clients' Self-Monitoring Logs (Alcohol: Client Handout 3.2; Drug: Client Handout 3.3)

Like Session 3, Session 4 begins with a discussion of the self-monitoring logs, but during this session the discussion focuses on whether any high-risk situations occurred since the last session and how clients handled them.

Personalized Feedback about Changes: Discussion of Comparative Personalized Feedback about Changes in Alcohol or Drug Use Over Treatment (Client Handouts 4.3 and 4.4, Respectively)

As the series of semistructured sessions is drawing to a close, clients are provided with feedback on their progress in the form of a comparison of their drinking or drug use prior to treatment with their use during treatment. In Session 1 clients were given a personalized feedback summary (i.e., Alcohol: Client Handout 4.1; Drug: Client Handout 4.2) based on their reports of their alcohol or drug use at the assessment. Reports of clients' alcohol and drug use during treatment come from their reports on their self-monitoring logs (Client Handouts 3.2 and 3.3, respectively). The reports of alcohol or drug use from the self-monitoring logs are compared with those prior to treatment. Examples of comparative alcohol and drug use feedback (90 days prior to treatment compared with the time from the assessment through Session 3) are shown in Client Handouts 4.3 and 4.4, respectively.

Comparative feedback is a motivational tool that allows therapists to have clients evaluate their own progress over treatment and give voice to changes they have made (e.g., *This graph shows your alcohol or drug use from before treatment to now. What about the graph stands out?*"). If progress has occurred, clients can be asked how they accomplished the change and how they feel about the changes they have made (i.e., giving voice to their change). If little or no change has occurred, then the comparison feedback graph sets the stage for a discussion of obstacles and what the next steps might be, again done in a motivationally enhancing manner by having clients reflect on their lack of change and where they want to go.

Comparative Goal Evaluation: Assessment and Session 3 (Abstinence: Client Handout 3.4; Low-Risk Limited Drinking: Client Handout 3.5)

The next topic in Session 4 is for clients to describe what they put down on their second goal evaluation and to compare it to their first goal evaluation. They are asked what, if anything, has changed and to describe what contributed to the change.

Decisional Balance Exercise Revisited (Client Handout 3.1)

For this discussion, the therapist revisits the decisional balance exercise that clients completed in Session 1. Clients are asked whether there are new things that should be added or changed. Important questions to ask include, *"Let's look at the decisional balance exercise you completed at the start of treatment. Are there any new good or less good things that you did not identify earlier?"* and *"Have any of the original good or less good things proved to be different from what you expected, and why?"* It is not unusual to hear clients say that changing was not as difficult as they expected it to be or to mention an unexpected benefit of changing (e.g., feeling more relaxed).

BSCQ Changes: Comparison of the High-Risk Profiles of Alcohol or Drug Use Completed at Assessment (Client Handout 4.7) and Session 3 (Client Handout 4.9)

In this part of the session, the therapist presents clients with comparative feedback on the BSCQ showing their changes (i.e., from assessment to Session 3) in confidence that they could resist the urge to drink heavily or to use drugs in different situations (Client Handout 4.9). When we observe increased confidence on the BSCQ profiles, we ask clients to explain what contributed to their increased confidence. In this way, clients are giving voice to changes that they have made. In turn, this discussion allows therapists an opportunity to reinforce clients' successes.

Discussion of the Implementation of New Options and Action Plans to Deal with High-Risk Trigger Situations

Because Session 4 for many clients will be their last session, a focus on maintenance of change is important. This can be done by reviewing how effective clients' options and action plans have been in terms of avoiding or dealing with high-risk situations since the last session, as well as what plans clients have developed should they encounter a setback or slip.

Where Are You Now Scale Readministered (Client Handout 3.6)

Once again, the client is asked to complete the Where Are You Now Scale. The new rating is discussed and compared with the ratings at the assessment and at Session 2. Because most clients will have improved somewhat, a good question to ask is, *"How did you get from where you were when you started treatment to where you are now, and how do you feel about the change?"*

Request for Additional Sessions (Client Handout 4.10)

Typically, the Request for Additional Sessions form is discussed near the end of this session. However, if a client is not making changes, a good jumping-off point is to discuss this form after a discussion of any comparison exercise that demonstrates a lack of substantial progress over the course of treatment (e.g., Where Are You Now Scale). Clients not requesting additional sessions can be reminded that the therapist will make an aftercare phone call about 1 month after the last session to see how they have been doing and that at that time clients can request further sessions if they have concerns or further problems. If clients request additional sessions, the therapist discusses this and the objectives for the additional sessions and then schedules the next appointment. The additional sessions and aftercare contact allow flexibility and individualization of treatment as needed for clients. In this regard, in the study that compared the GSC intervention in a group versus an individual format, at the 1-year follow-up 64% of those interviewed felt that the aftercare calls were helpful, and 23% would have liked more calls (L. C. Sobell et al., 2009).

End of Session: Wrap-Up and What Stood Out

Clients are asked, *"What stood out about today's session?"*

SUMMARY

This chapter presented a detailed description of how to conduct GSC using an individual-therapy format. Using a motivational interviewing style, therapists lead clients through the major components of the intervention. These components include receiving feedback based on information provided at the assessment, establishing goals, evaluating motivation using the decisional balance exercise, conducting a functional analysis of factors setting the occasion for and following problematic substance use, and applying a problem-solving approach to develop plans for change. With therapists' assistance, clients take major responsibility for developing a basic understanding of their problem and the basis of their motivation for change and for generating and implementing a reasonable plan for change.

Objectives, Procedures, Client Handouts, and Clinical Guidelines and Dialogues
Individual Session 1

SESSION OBJECTIVES

- Follow up on any inquiries from the assessment.
- Review client's progress.
- Review and discuss client's goal evaluation; provide guidelines or information on contraindications for use, if appropriate.
- Review self-monitoring logs with respect to the client's goal.
- Provide client with personalized feedback based on the assessment.
- Give homework and instructions for Session 2.

PRIOR TO SESSION

- Review assessment information; identify any areas needing further information or clarification.
- Prepare feedback based on assessment information.
- Get new homework for client (Client Handouts 4.5 and 4.6).

SESSION PROCEDURES

- Introduce session.
- Review and discuss client's completed self-monitoring log; copy or record data.
- Review and discuss client's understanding of homework reading on Identifying Triggers exercise.
- Give client personalized feedback from assessment and discuss.
- Review and discuss completed goal evaluation form with client.
- Review and discuss completed decisional balance exercise with client.
- Ask client the five-million-dollar question and affirm that changing is a choice.
- End session: What stood out today about session; remind them to do homework; schedule next session.

CLIENT HANDOUTS

- Reading: Identifying Triggers (Client Handout 4.5)
- Exercise: Identifying Triggers (Client Handout 4.6)

COMPLETE BEFORE SESSION 2

- Review and make session notes.
- Prepare the BSCQ graphs for Session 2 based on the Assessment BSCQ.

(cont.)

CLINICAL GUIDELINES AND DIALOGUES FOR THERAPISTS CONDUCTING
INDIVIDUAL THERAPY SESSION 1

Self-Monitoring and Goal Evaluations

Therapist (T): *"How did your week go?"*

Note to Therapist: Focus the discussion on major events or patterns. Do not have clients do a day-by-day discussion of their week. Use the next question as a jumping-off point to discuss what clients put down on their self-monitoring logs. The therapist can begin by saying, *"Let's take a look at what you put down on your self-monitoring log."*

Note to Therapist: This section is for clients who chose an abstinence goal (includes clients with drug problems).

T: *"Now, let's take a look at your goal evaluation form."* (Client Handout 3.4)

T: *"What did you put down for the importance of your goal? Why did you select a* [**insert # they gave**] *rather than a* [**lower #**]*?"*

T: *"What did you put down for how confident you are in achieving your goal? Why did you select a* [**insert # client gave**] *rather than a* [**lower #**]*?"*

T: (if appropriate) *"So, it sounds like you definitely want to stop using alcohol or drugs. What, if anything, might get in your way?"*

Note to Therapist: This section is for clients who selected a low-risk limited drinking goal and for whom there were no contraindications. Let clients say what goal they selected—abstinence or low-risk drinking.

T: *"Now, let's take a look at your goal evaluation form."* (Client Handout 3.5)

T: *"Tell me what goal you selected."*

Possible Questions

T: *"How did you arrive at your goal?"*

T: *"How realistic is this goal for you?"*

Explain the Low-Risk Limited Drinking Guidelines

T: *"We have some guidelines for low-risk limited drinking that I would like to review with you. One of the guidelines is referred to as a 3/4 rule. We recommend that you have no more than 3 drinks per day on no more than 4 days per week, that you do not drink in high-risk situations, and that you drink at a rate of no more than one drink per hour."*

Note to Therapist: Use only if client's goal is within the recommended guidelines.

T: *"So, as you can see, your goal is within our recommended limits."*

Note to Therapist: Use only if client's goal exceeds the recommended guidelines.

T: *"Your goal is over our recommended low-risk limited drinking guidelines. Now that we've gone over the guidelines, how do you view your goal?"*

(cont.)

Note to Therapist: The client may change the goal to be within the guidelines. If the client still chooses a goal that exceeds the guidelines, the therapist can say, *"Although your goal is more than our recommendation, it is less than what you were averaging before coming into treatment. How would you see yourself further reducing your drinking over the next few months?"*

T: *"What did you put down for the circumstances under which you would not drink and the situations in which it was safer for you to drink in a limited manner?"*

T: *"Why do you think we have people select their own goal?"*

T: *"Now, let's take a look at your importance and confidence ratings."*

T: *"What did you put down for the importance of your goal? Why did you select a* [**insert # client gave**] *rather than a* [**lower #**]*?"*

T: *"What did you put down for how confident you are in achieving your goal? Why did you select a* [**insert # client gave**] *rather than a* [**lower #**]*?"*

T: (if appropriate) *"So, it sounds like changing your drinking is very important to you right now. What, if anything, might get in your way?"*

Note to Therapist: With clients who are ambivalent about their goal, the therapist can ask, *"On the one hand it sounds like your goal is important and you want to change, but on the other hand you are concerned about many other things going on in your life, like your career and your family, that are also priorities for you right now. If you don't make some changes now, what effect do you think your* [**insert substance name**] *use would have on your life in the next year?"*
The therapist might follow with, *"What one thing do you think it would take for you to stop using* [**insert substance name**] *right now?"*

Providing Clients with Feedback from Their Assessment Data

T: *"If you remember, at the assessment session I asked you many questions and you filled out some forms about your alcohol or drug use, including a calendar showing your alcohol or drug use over the past few months. We have taken this information and prepared a personalized feedback summary for you so you can see where your alcohol [or drug] use fits in compared with that of others. This provides people with information that allows them to make more informed decisions about changing."*

Note to Therapist: Show the client a copy of the feedback summary that was prepared (Alcohol: Client Handout 4.3; Drug: Client Handout 4.4).

T: *"So you reported drinking, on average* [**insert #**] *drinks per week. On this graph, where does that put you in terms of all men/women who drink?"*

T: *"The bottom of this page is your AUDIT [or DAST-10] score, which reflects the severity of your reported alcohol [or drug] use (AUDIT: Client Handout 4.1; DAST-10: Client Handout 4.2)."*

Note to Therapist: If clients are surprised about the severity level of their alcohol or drug use on the AUDIT or DAST-10, the therapist can say, *"Well, let's look at your answers to some of the questions."*

Decisional Balance Exercise (Client Handout 3.1)

T: *"Last week we also asked you to complete and bring back to this session a decisional balance exercise. What did you get out of the exercise?"*

(cont.)

Probe and discuss using open-ended questions, followed by reflections and, when appropriate, summary statements. Answers should include some mention of the following.

T: *"This exercise can help you organize and evaluate the good things and less good things about your alcohol or drug use. It also helps you to see the full range of good and less good things."*

T: *"Tell me about what you listed as the good things about your [**insert substance name**] use."*

T: *"Now, what are the less good things?"*

T: *"Okay, what did you list as the good things and less good things about changing?"*

Note to Therapist: It is important for the client to be aware of the possible costs of changing, as that sets the stage for planning how to avoid or minimize those costs.

The Five-Million-Dollar Question
(LAST PART OF DECISIONAL BALANCE EXERCISE, CLIENT HANDOUT 3.1)

T: *"Now that we've discussed the good things and less good things about your alcohol or drug use, what would it take for you to tip the scale and change your behavior* **right now***? What if I offered you $5 million to change your alcohol or drug use for just for one day?"*

Because most clients respond affirmatively, the therapist could ask, *"So what does that tell you?"* The therapist could then say, *"Well, I don't have $5 million, but what we are asking you to think about is what your personal price is for changing."*
Note to Therapist: The idea is that changing is a choice that people can make, although it might be a difficult choice. Once a client recognizes that changing is a choice, then the question becomes what will it take in order to make that choice.

Explaining Identifying Triggers Reading and Exercise
(CLIENT HANDOUTS 4.5 AND 4.6, RESPECTIVELY)

T: *"Let us switch gears and look at the next homework assignment."*

T: *"I've noticed that you've mentioned some situations in which you feel as though your alcohol or drug use has caused you some problems, and that leads us into the next homework, which is about identifying triggers. There are two parts to this homework, a short reading and then the Identifying Triggers exercise. You should read the reading first, and then do the exercise, which involves identifying your two highest risk situations for alcohol or drug use in the past year. We would like you to describe the triggers in detail, such as where and when they take place and the consequences that follow alcohol or drug use. How to complete the exercise is explained at the beginning of the handout. Completing this homework and bringing it to the next session gives us an opportunity to talk more about these high-risk trigger situations and examine why they've been a problem for you."*

End of Session: What Stood Out

T: *"We talked about many things today. What stood out for you?"*

Objectives, Procedures, Client Handouts, and Clinical Guidelines and Dialogues
Individual Session 2

SESSION OBJECTIVES

- Review client's progress.
- Identify high-risk situations for client based on homework and BSCQ.
- Give homework and instructions for Session 3.

PRIOR TO SESSION

- Prepare and have BSCQ personalized feedback profile ready for client based on the assessment BSCQ.
- Get new homework for client (Client Handout 4.8).

SESSION PROCEDURES

- Introduce session.
- Review and discuss client's completed self-monitoring log; copy or record data.
- Review and discuss client's answers to Identifying Triggers homework exercise.
- Give client BSCQ feedback profile (Client Handout 4.7) and discuss relationship to Identifying Triggers homework answers.
- Have client complete Where Are You Now Scale (Client Handout 3.6) and compare with assessment answer on same form.
- End session: Ask what stood out about session, schedule next session, and remind client to do homework.

CLIENT HANDOUTS

- Exercise: Developing Options and Action Plans (Client Handout 4.8)
- Have the client's *Where Are You Now Scale* to use in this session

COMPLETE BEFORE TREATMENT SESSION 3

- Review and make session notes.

(cont.)

CLINICAL GUIDELINES AND DIALOGUES FOR THERAPISTS CONDUCTING INDIVIDUAL THERAPY SESSION 2

Review Self-Monitoring Logs

Therapist (T): *"How have things been since our last session?"* [The intent is to get clients to discuss their self-monitoring logs.]

The therapist can begin by saying, *"Let's take a look at what you put down on your self-monitoring logs since our last session."*

Note to Therapist: Remember to look for the big picture rather than a day-by-day report. For this and subsequent sessions, the therapist should reflect what the client says and how the client's week went. For example, the therapist could reflect, *"It sounds like this was a good week for you as you made some significant changes since last session. How do you feel about these changes?"* or *"It sounds like you are still struggling a bit with not drinking or using drugs."*

Discuss Identifying Triggers Reading and Exercise
(Client Handouts 4.5 and 4.6, Respectively)

T: *"Let's take a look at the reading and homework on identifying triggers that you took home last week."* (Reading: Client Handout 4.5; Exercise: Client Handout 4.6)

T: *"The reading for this week described changing as climbing a mountain. What did you get out of the reading?"*

If the client understands the concept of Mt. Change, then the therapist can say, *"It sounds like you understood what we were trying to communicate with this diagram. Although it would be nice to wake up tomorrow and your alcohol or drug use is no longer a concern, realistically most people experience some bumps in the road. What we would like you to do is to view a slip or lapse as a learning experience and move on."*

If the client does not seem to understand the concept of Mt. Change, then the therapist can say, *"This reading was intended to help you adopt a realistic, long-term perspective on changing your alcohol or drug use. Although it would be nice to change overnight, for some people it is a slower process."*

Note to Therapist: The important points from the reading are taking a realistic perspective on change (i.e., Mt. Change) and the importance of viewing slips as learning experiences. When discussing the possibility of slips, it is also essential that the therapist not convey a self-fulfilling prophecy to the client (i.e., that slips will occur). A good way of presenting the concept that also avoids such a prophecy is as a fire drill. Thus the client can be asked, *"Why do you think we have fire drills in school?"* Clients will almost always come up with the obvious reason that you are better prepared if a fire occurs.

The therapist can follow this with, *"That's the same idea here. Hopefully you won't have any slips, but it makes sense to be prepared in case they do happen. If a slip or lapse occurs, the important thing is to interrupt it as soon as possible, see what you can learn from it, and get back on track. To learn from this experience, you can ask yourself, 'What was different about this situation?' or `How can I deal with this situation differently next time?'"*

T: *"Now let's take a look at what you put down for your two high-risk trigger situations for alcohol or drug use. Tell me a bit about those situations."*

(cont.)

Note to Therapist: Have clients discuss what they put down. The therapist reflects what the client says, but because the trigger situations are critical in terms of the change process, the therapist needs to fully explore these situations with the client.

Sample Responses to the Client's Identified Triggers

- *"It looks like one high-risk situation for you is being alone and having drugs available to you."*
- *"So it sounds like you are having trouble balancing raising your kids and your career and at the end of the day you need something to cope."*
- *"Let me see if I understand what you are meaning about that second situation. It sounds like you're saying a trigger can happen when you have some free time and are bored."*

REVIEW BRIEF SITUATIONAL CONFIDENCE QUESTIONNAIRE

T: *"One of the things you did at the assessment was to complete a questionnaire called the Brief Situational Confidence Questionnaire. It asked you about your ability to resist the urge to drink heavily or use drugs in eight common high-risk situations. I graphed your confidence levels in those situations, and I have highlighted the three situations in which you indicated you were least confident in your ability to resist the urge to drink heavily or use drugs. What stands out to you about this graph?"*

Note to Therapist: The goal is to have clients give voice to the fact that risk varies with situations and that some situations are particularly high risk for them. It is then explained to clients that sometimes it is easier to remember their high-risk situations by referring to them using a shorthand label. Table 4.2 presents several types of BSCQ profiles to which we have given shorthand names (e.g., Good Times; Negative Affective; Testing Personal Control) that can be easily remembered. The therapist then goes on to ask clients to relate their BSCQ profile to their answers on the Identifying Triggers exercise. We have found that in almost all cases the client's two personal high-risk trigger situations are similar to what is shown in their generic BSCQ profile.

T: *"Tell me what you see in terms of how your profile of high-risk situations compares with the two high-risk situations you identified in the Identifying Triggers exercise we just discussed."*

Reflect what the client says here: *"What I hear you saying is that the most problematic situations are those in which you experience negative emotions."*

If the client's two high-risk situations and generic BSCQ profile are similar, then the therapist can say, *"Your profile provides a shorthand of what situations you should be on guard for in the coming weeks. For example, between now and the next session, which of these general situations do you see yourself possibly encountering?"*

Revisit the Where Are You Now Scale

T: *"When you first came in, we asked you to rate how serious you thought your alcohol or drug use was on a 10-point scale. On that same scale, where 1 = the most serious concern and 10 = no longer a concern, how would rate your alcohol or drug use today?"*

T: *"Do you remember what number characterized where you were at the assessment interview on this scale? [***Client answers***] How did you go from a [***# at Assessment***] to a [***# now***]?"*

(cont.)

Note to Therapist: The Where Are You Now Scale is a motivational interviewing technique that allows therapists to ask clients to give voice to changes they have made. For a client who has not changed, the therapist can say, *"What would you need to do to move up a number or two?"* or *"What kinds of things have gotten in the way of your changing?"*

Introduce Homework Exercise: Developing New Options and Action Plans (Client Handout 4.8)

T: *"The next homework exercise asks you to develop new options and action plans for the two high-risk trigger situations in today's exercise. What we would like you to do is to take these two high-risk trigger situations and come up with some new options and then evaluate how well they might work to help you resist using alcohol or drugs. After you have developed the options, evaluate them and decide which is your best one. Then develop a plan of action for how to put the option into practice. When making action plans, try to break them down into several smaller steps so it is easier to see your progress. The exercise should take about 10 minutes to complete."*

End of Session: What Stood Out

T: *"We talked about many things today. What stood out for you?"*

Objectives, Procedures, Client Handouts, and Clinical Guidelines and Dialogues
Individual Session 3

SESSION OBJECTIVES

- Review client's progress.
- Discuss client's change plans.

PRIOR TO SESSION

- Get new homework for clients.
    Request for Additional Sessions form (Client Handout 4.10)
    Goal evaluation form (Client Handout 3.4 for members with an abstinence goal; Client Handout 3.5 for members with a low-risk limited drinking goal)
- Get a BSCQ form (Appendix D) for client to complete in session

SESSION PROCEDURES

- Introduce session.
- Review and discuss client's completed self-monitoring log; copy or record data.
- Have client complete new BSCQ in session (second administration).
- Review and discuss client's answers to the Developing New Options and Action Plans homework exercise (Client Handout 4.8).
- Discuss possible opportunities for testing options before Session 4.
- End session: Ask what stood out about session, schedule next session, remind client to do homework.

CLIENT HANDOUTS

- Give client Request for Additional Sessions form (Client Handout 4.10) as homework
- Give client goal evaluation form (Abstinence: Client Handout 3.4; Low-Risk Limited Drinking: Client Handout 3.5) as homework
- BSCQ form (Appendix D) to be completed in session

COMPLETE BEFORE TREATMENT SESSION 4

- Review and make session notes.
- Prepare personalized comparative BSCQ profile (assessment and Session 3) of the client's high-risk situations for alcohol or drug use (Client Handout 4.9).
- Prepare a personalized comparative (Assessment to Session 3) feedback form of the client's alcohol or drug use (Alcohol: Client Handout 4.3; Drug: Client Handout 4.4).

(cont.)

CLINICAL GUIDELINES AND DIALOGUES FOR THERAPISTS CONDUCTING INDIVIDUAL THERAPY SESSION 3

Review Self-Monitoring Logs

T: *"How have things been since our last session?"* [Here the therapist is trying to get the client to discuss his or her self-monitoring logs. The therapist can begin by saying, *"Let's take a look at what you put down on your self-monitoring logs this week."*

Note to Therapist: Remember to keep the discussion to the main features of the log, rather than having a day-by-day description. Have clients relate the recent drinking or drug use to their goal.

Discuss Developing New Options and Actions Plans Homework (Client Handout 4.8)

T: *"The homework we asked you to complete for this session asked you to develop new options and action plans for the two high-risk trigger situations you identified last week. Let's start by discussing the various options you thought of for each trigger and then which action plan makes the most sense for you to implement and why."*

Note to Therapist: Use open-ended questions, reflections, and summary statements to explore the client's options and action plans and their feasibility. Emphasize the need to break the action plans into small steps when possible.

T: *"What situations can you anticipate occurring between now and your next session in which you could put into practice your options and action plans?"*

In-Session Assignment

Give the client another BSCQ to complete (Appendix D)

T: *"This is another copy of a form that you filled out at the assessment, the Brief Situational Confidence Questionnaire. What we would like you to do is to fill it out again, reflecting how you feel today. We will discuss it at next week's session."*

Homework Assignments for Session 4

Give the client another goal evaluation form (Client Handout 3.4 for clients with an abstinence goal; Client Handout 3.5 for clients with a low-risk limited drinking goal)

T: *"Your homework for next week is to fill out two more forms. The first is another goal statement, like the first one you completed at the assessment session. Fill it out and bring it to the next session."*

T: *"As was mentioned at the assessment, next week will be our last group session. Some people will feel they do not need any additional sessions, as they have made enough progress, whereas others will want to continue in treatment. On this form you can indicate whether you want additional sessions and, if so, how many and what you would like to accomplish."*

End of Session: What Stood Out

T: *"We talked about many things today. What stood out for you?"*

Objectives, Procedures, Client Handouts, and Clinical Guidelines and Dialogues
Individual Session 4

SESSION OBJECTIVES

- Review client's progress.
- Revisit and review client's motivation and goal.
- Discuss end of treatment and aftercare call or schedule further sessions.

PRIOR TO SESSION

- Prepare BSCQ comparison profiles from the assessment and Session 3 (Client Handout 4.9).
- Prepare personalized comparative feedback (assessment to Session 3) for Alcohol Use (Client Handout 4.3) or Drug Use (Client Handout 4.4).
- Have the Where Are You Now Scale for the client to complete again (Client Handout 3.6).

SESSION PROCEDURES

- Introduce session.
- Review and discuss client's completed self-monitoring log in relation to goal; copy or record data.
- Discuss opportunities for testing options since last session and the outcomes.
- Give client personalized feedback comparison (assessment to Session 3) of his or her alcohol use (Client Handout 4.3) or drug use (Client Handout 4.4) and discuss.
- Revisit goal, revise if necessary.
- Revisit decisional balance exercise, revise if necessary.
- Give client BSCQ comparison (Client Handout 4.9) of assessment and Session 3 answers and discuss.
- Revisit and review client's understanding of Identifying Triggers reading related to Mt. Change and taking a realistic, long-term perspective on change.
- Have client complete Where Are You Now Scale and compare it with his or her assessment and Session 2 answers (Client Handout 3.6).
- Discuss Request for Additional Sessions form (Client Handout 4.10) completed as homework by client.
- Ensure that clients know how to contact the program if they need further treatment. Also, mention that you will call them in about a month after their last session to inquire about their progress, to support their changes, and to schedule additional sessions if needed.
- End session: Ask what stood out about the session.
- Make session notes.

(cont.)

CLINICAL GUIDELINES AND DIALOGUES FOR THERAPISTS CONDUCTING
INDIVIDUAL THERAPY SESSION 4

Review Self-Monitoring Logs

Therapist (T): *"How have things been since our last session?"* [Because the client is now familiar with the procedure of starting by discussing the self-monitoring logs, the therapist asks the client to discuss his or her self-monitoring logs.]

The therapist can begin by saying, *"Let's take a look at what you put down on your self-monitoring logs."*

Note to Therapist: If major changes have occurred or the client successfully handled a difficult situation and did not use, the therapist can have the client give voice to the changes.

T: *"That's two weeks with no drinking, which is a big change for you. How were you able to do that?"* The client's response can be followed by a reflection from the therapist. For example, *"So by letting your friends know what you were trying to do, you found they were helpful and you were able to stop using. How do you feel about that change?"*

Revisiting Alcohol or Drug Use from Assessment to Session 3

Give clients their personalized feedback comparison of their alcohol use (Client Handout 4.3) or drug use (Client Handout 4.4) from the assessment to Session 3. This feedback allows clients to give voice to changes they made in their alcohol or drug use rather than having the therapist tell them about the changes.

Alcohol Clients

T: *"The information you provided about your drinking when you first came in and over the course of treatment is shown in this graph. The first graph compares how frequently (% of days) you drank during the 90 days preceding your treatment and during the time you have been in the program. In looking at this graph, how would you say your drinking has changed?"*

T: *"The second graph compares how much you drank on days when you did drink during the 90 days preceding your treatment and during the time you have been in the program. In looking at this graph, how would you say your drinking has changed?"*

Drug Clients

T: *"The information you provided about your drug use when you first came in and during the time you have been in treatment is shown in this graph. This graph compares how frequently (% of days) you used drugs during the 90 days preceding your treatment and during the time you have been in the program. In looking at this graph, how would you say your drug use has changed?"*

(cont.)

Comparative Goal Evaluations

Goal Evaluation: Abstinence (Client Handout 3.4)

T: *"If you remember, when you first came in you rated the importance of and your confidence in not using alcohol or drugs. Part of your homework for this week was to fill out another goal evaluation form. Let's take a look at your new evaluation and compare it with the goal evaluation you completed when you first came in. How have your importance and confidence ratings changed, and what led to those changes?"*

Goal Evaluation: Goal Choice (Client Handout 3.5)

T: *"If you remember, when you first came in you selected a goal, and part of the homework for this week was to fill out that form again. How has it changed, if at all, and why?"*

T: *"How have your importance and confidence ratings changed, and what led to those changes?"*

Decisional Balance Revisited from Session 1

Note to Therapist: Refer back to the first decisional balance exercise with the client (Client Handout 3.1)

Possible Questions

T: *"Let's look at the decisional balance exercise you completed at the start of treatment. Are there any new good or less good things that you did not identify earlier?"*

T: *"Have any of the original good or less good things proved to be different from what you expected, and why?"* [Often clients will report that anticipated negative consequences of changing did not occur after all.]

Changes in Brief Situational Confidence Questionnaires

Give clients the BSCQ comparison profiles (Client Handout 4.9) of their assessment and Session 3 answers.

T: *"Let's look at the second Brief Situational Confidence Questionnaire you completed last week and compare it to the one you filled out at the assessment. What I have done is to combine both profiles on one sheet for you. What changes do you notice in your ability to resist the urge to drink heavily or to use drugs in these eight different high-risk situations?"* [Client answers] *"What led to changes in your confidence in these situations?"*

Implementation of Options

T: *"What situations came up since the last session in which you were able to put one of your action plans to work? How did it turn out?"*

(cont.)

Mt. Change Revisited

T: *"Based on our previous discussions, what does taking a realistic perspective on change mean to you?"*

Note to Therapist: Look for the fact that change can be slow, but that it is important to learn from slips and keep going.

Where Are You Now Scale Revisited (Client Handout 3.6)

T: *"When you first came in, and again at the second session, I asked you to rate how serious you thought your alcohol or drug use was on a 10-point scale. How would you rate your alcohol or drug use today on that same scale where 1 = the most serious concern and 10 = no longer a concern? Do you remember what you said on the two previous occasions? [Client answers] How did you get from a [# at assessment] to a [# now]?"*

Review Request for Additional Sessions Form (Client Handout 4.10)

T: "Before we wrap up, last week I gave you a Request for Additional Sessions form to fill out and bring in today. Let's take a look at what you put down."

Note to Therapist: If the client requests additional sessions, schedule an appointment and note how many extra sessions were requested and why. If the client does not request additional sessions, remind him or her that you will call in 1 month to see how he or she is doing.

End of Session: What Stood Out

T: *"We talked about many things today. What stood out for you?"*

Personalized Feedback: Where Does Your Alcohol Use Fit In?
Individual and Group Session 1

THINKING ABOUT CHANGING?

Based on your answers to questionnaires you completed earlier, we have prepared a **personalized summary** of your **ALCOHOL USE**. These include:

1. **A graph showing how much men and women drink per week. Compare your alcohol use with that of others to see where you fit in.**

   You reported drinking on _____ % of the last 90 days.

   You reported drinking an average of _____ drinks per week.

2. **Your score on the AUDIT**, a questionnaire that evaluates the extent to which a person's alcohol use is a problem. **Where does your score fit in?**

3. **Consequences you reported that are related to your alcohol use.**

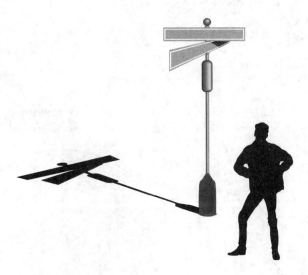

(cont.)

Number of Drinks Consumed in a Week
By Adults Surveyed in the United States*

Where Does Your Drinking Fit In?

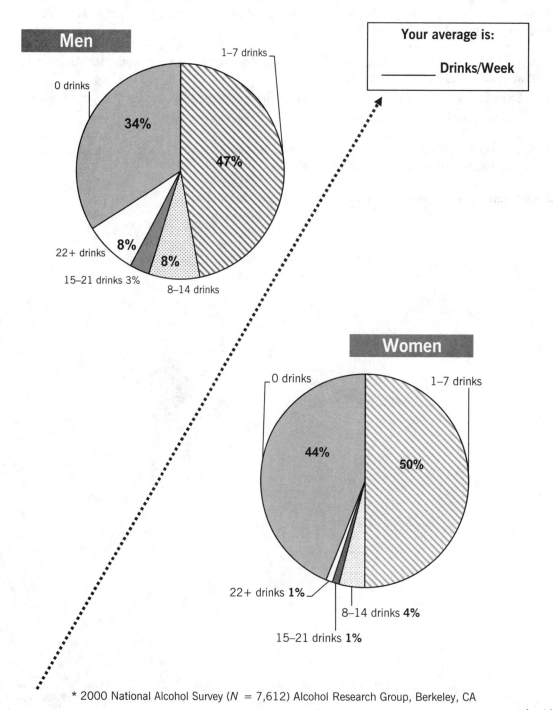

Your average is:

_____ **Drinks/Week**

Men

0 drinks — **34%**

1–7 drinks — **47%**

22+ drinks — **8%**

15–21 drinks 3%

8–14 drinks — **8%**

Women

0 drinks — **44%**

1–7 drinks — **50%**

22+ drinks **1%**

8–14 drinks **4%**

15–21 drinks **1%**

* 2000 National Alcohol Survey (*N* = 7,612) Alcohol Research Group, Berkeley, CA

(cont.)

116

Where Does Your ALCOHOL Use Fit In?

The AUDIT questionnaire was developed by the World Health Organization to evaluate a person's use of alcohol and the extent to which drinking is a problem for them. Below is your AUDIT score, which is based on materials you filled out earlier. Higher scores typically reflect more serious problems.

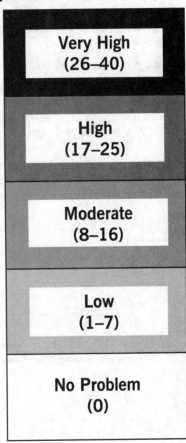

Where Do You Fit In?
Your AUDIT Score is

_____

Personalized Feedback: Where Does Your Drug Use Fit In?
Individual and Group Therapy Session 1

THINKING ABOUT CHANGING?

The following information relates to your use of _____

Primary Drug

Based on your answers to questionnaires you completed earlier, we have prepared a **personalized summary** of your **DRUG USE**. These include:

1. **A graph showing how many people have used your primary drug in the past year, past month, and lifetime.**

   Compare your drug use with that of others to see where you fit in.

   You reported using drugs on _____ % of days in the last 3 months.

2. **Your score on the DAST**, a questionnaire that evaluates the extent to which a person's drug use is a problem. **Where does your score fit in?**

3. **Consequences you reported that are related to your drug use.**

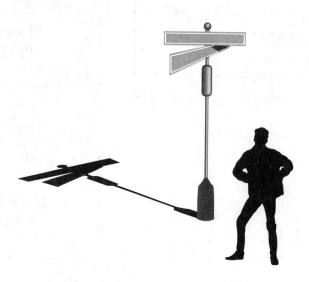

Cocaine and Crack Use by Persons
12 Years and Older in the United States*

Where Do You Fit In?

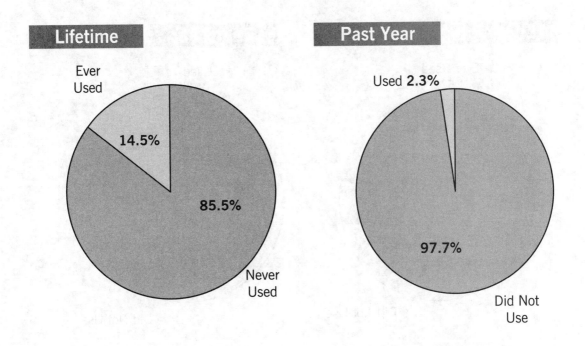

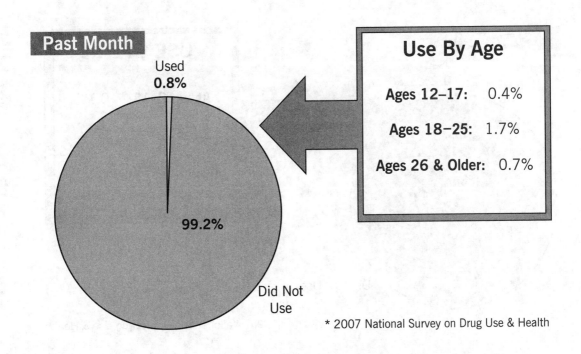

Use By Age

Ages 12–17: 0.4%

Ages 18–25: 1.7%

Ages 26 & Older: 0.7%

* 2007 National Survey on Drug Use & Health

119

Crack Use by Persons
12 Years and Older in the United States*

Where Do You Fit In?

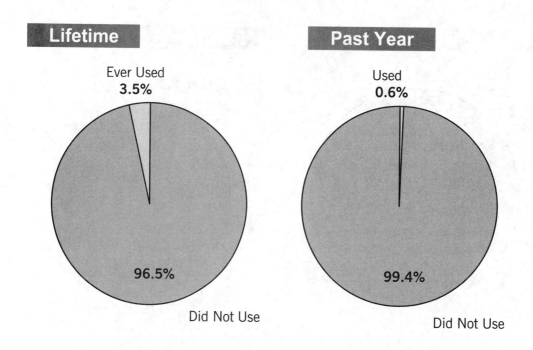

Lifetime

Ever Used
3.5%

96.5%

Did Not Use

Past Year

Used
0.6%

99.4%

Did Not Use

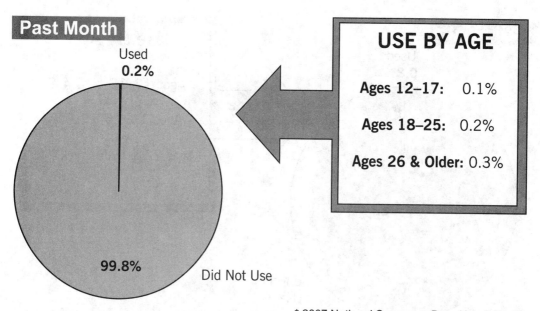

Past Month

Used
0.2%

99.8%

Did Not Use

USE BY AGE

Ages 12–17: 0.1%

Ages 18–25: 0.2%

Ages 26 & Older: 0.3%

* 2007 National Survey on Drug Use & Health

Hallucinogens Use by Persons
12 Years and Older in the United States*

Where Do You Fit In?

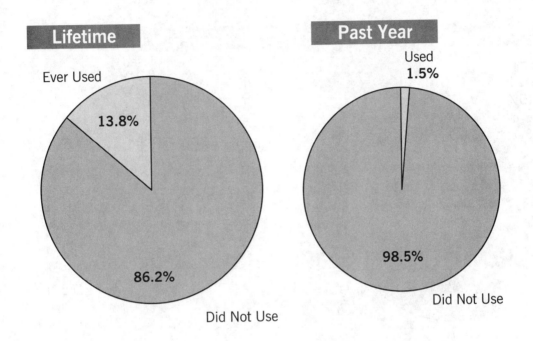

Lifetime

Ever Used
13.8%

86.2%

Did Not Use

Past Year

Used
1.5%

98.5%

Did Not Use

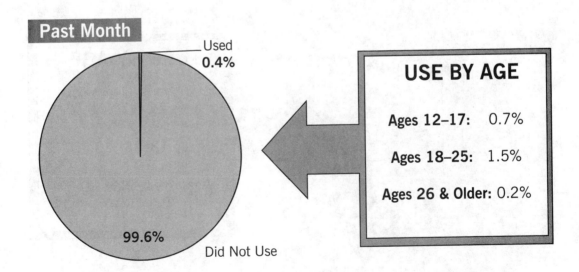

Past Month

Used
0.4%

99.6%

Did Not Use

USE BY AGE

Ages 12–17: 0.7%

Ages 18–25: 1.5%

Ages 26 & Older: 0.2%

* 2007 National Survey on Drug Use & Health

Heroin Use by Persons
12 Years and Older in the United States*

Where Do You Fit In?

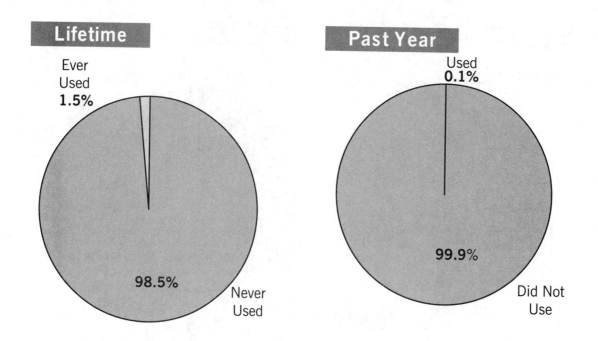

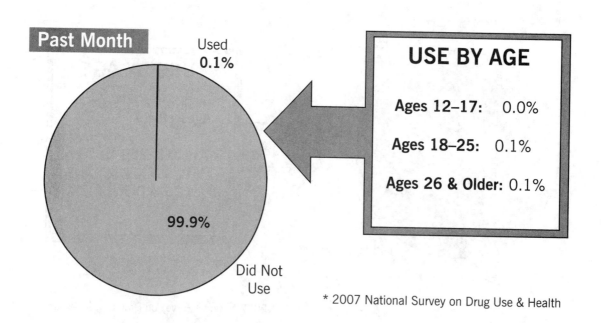

* 2007 National Survey on Drug Use & Health

Inhalant Use by Persons
12 Years and Older in the United States*

Where Do You Fit In?

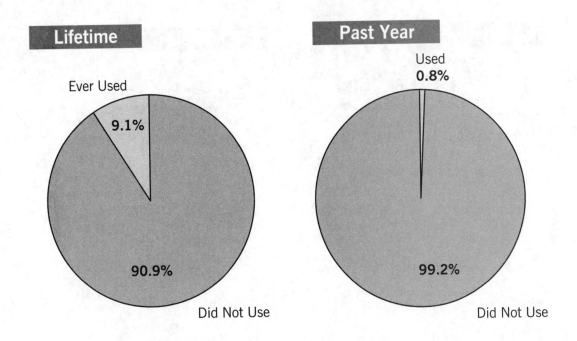

Lifetime

Ever Used

9.1%

90.9%

Did Not Use

Past Year

Used
0.8%

99.2%

Did Not Use

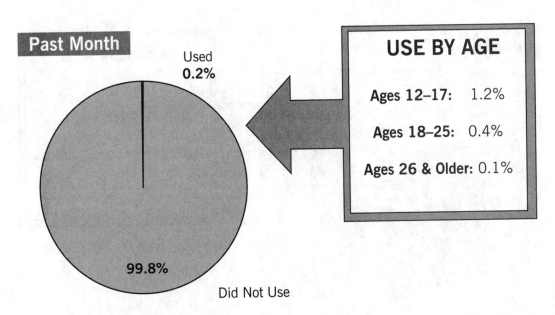

Past Month

Used
0.2%

99.8%

Did Not Use

USE BY AGE

Ages 12–17: 1.2%

Ages 18–25: 0.4%

Ages 26 & Older: 0.1%

* 2007 National Survey on Drug Use & Health

Cigarette Use by Persons
18 Years and Older in the United States*

Where Do You Fit In?

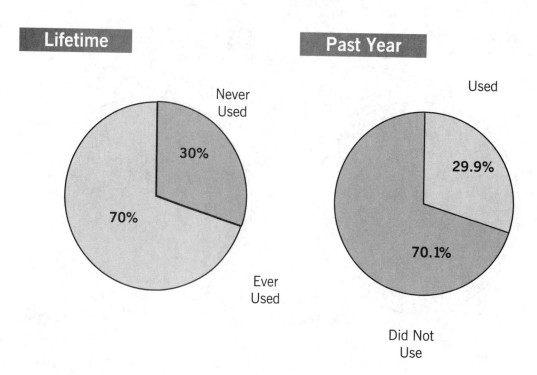

Lifetime

Never Used

30%

70%

Ever Used

Past Year

Used

29.9%

70.1%

Did Not Use

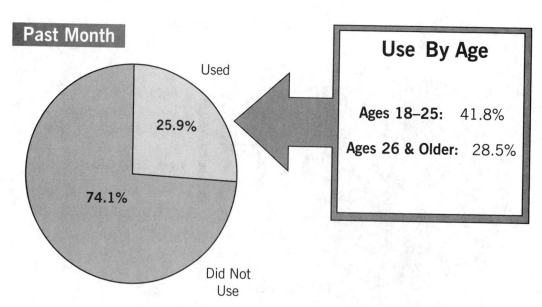

Past Month

Used

25.9%

74.1%

Did Not Use

Use By Age

Ages 18–25: 41.8%

Ages 26 & Older: 28.5%

* 2007 National Survey on Drug Use & Health

Marijuana and Hashish Use by Persons
12 Years and Older in the United States*

Where Do You Fit In?

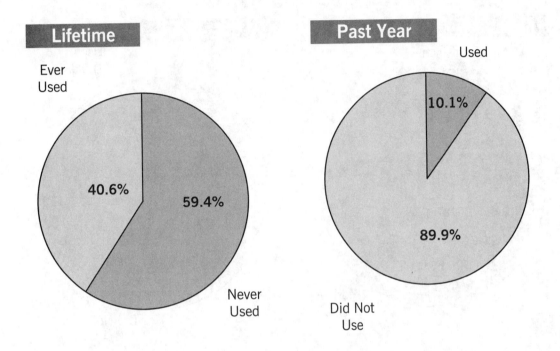

Lifetime

Ever
Used

40.6%

59.4%

Never
Used

Past Year

Used

10.1%

89.9%

Did Not
Use

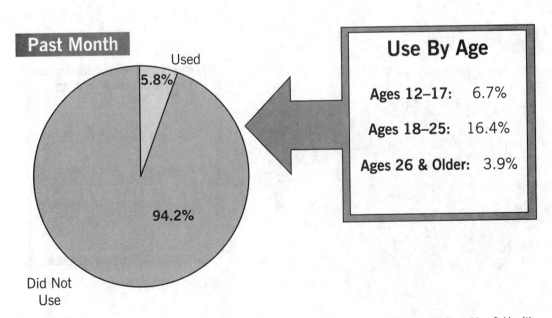

Past Month

Used

5.8%

94.2%

Did Not
Use

Use By Age

Ages 12–17: 6.7%

Ages 18–25: 16.4%

Ages 26 & Older: 3.9%

* 2007 National Survey on Drug Use & Health

125

Nonmedical Methamphetamine Use by Persons
12 Years and Older in the United States*

Where Do You Fit In?

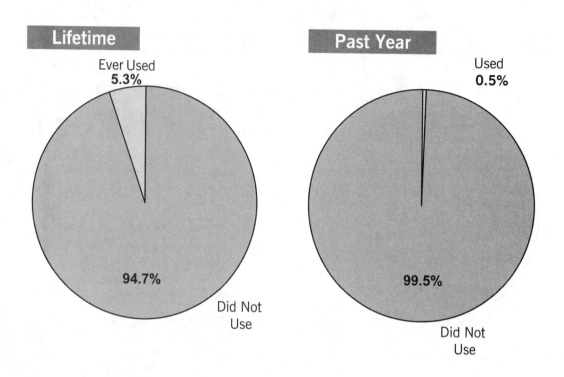

Lifetime

Ever Used
5.3%

94.7%

Did Not
Use

Past Year

Used
0.5%

99.5%

Did Not
Use

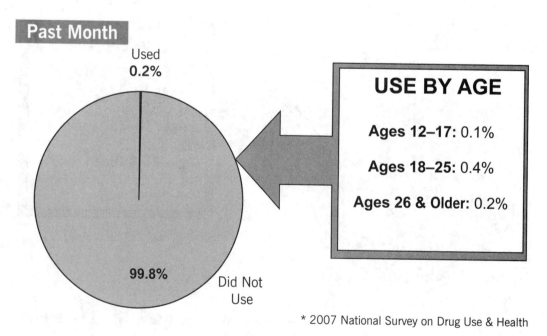

Past Month

Used
0.2%

99.8%

Did Not
Use

USE BY AGE

Ages 12–17: 0.1%

Ages 18–25: 0.4%

Ages 26 & Older: 0.2%

* 2007 National Survey on Drug Use & Health

Nonmedical OxyContin® Use by Persons 12 Years and Older in the United States*

Where Do You Fit In?

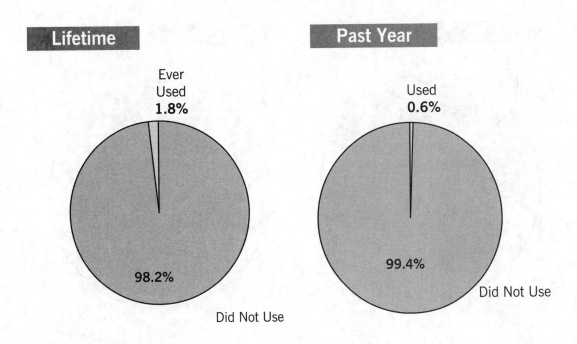

Lifetime

Ever
Used
1.8%

98.2%

Did Not Use

Past Year

Used
0.6%

99.4%

Did Not Use

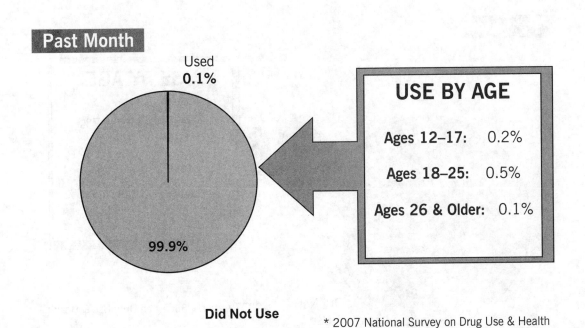

Past Month

Used
0.1%

99.9%

Did Not Use

USE BY AGE

Ages 12–17:   0.2%

Ages 18–25:   0.5%

Ages 26 & Older: 0.1%

* 2007 National Survey on Drug Use & Health

Nonmedical Use of Pain Relievers by Persons
12 Years and Older in the United States*

Where Do You Fit In?

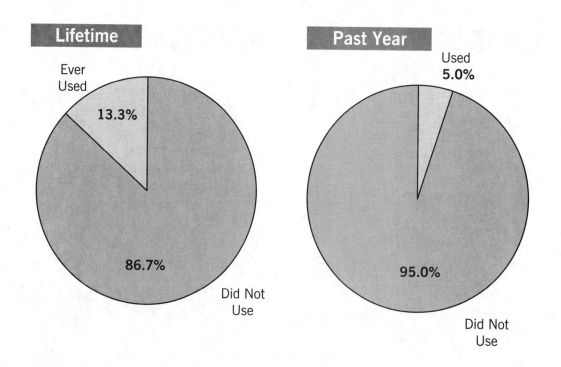

Lifetime

Ever Used

13.3%

86.7%

Did Not Use

Past Year

Used
5.0%

95.0%

Did Not Use

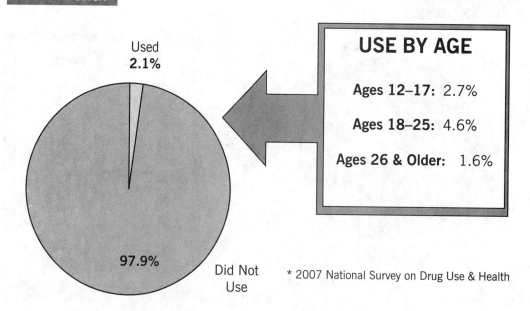

Past Month

Used
2.1%

97.9%

Did Not Use

USE BY AGE

Ages 12–17: 2.7%

Ages 18–25: 4.6%

Ages 26 & Older: 1.6%

* 2007 National Survey on Drug Use & Health

Nonmedical Sedative Use by Persons
12 Years and Older in the United States*

Where Do You Fit In?

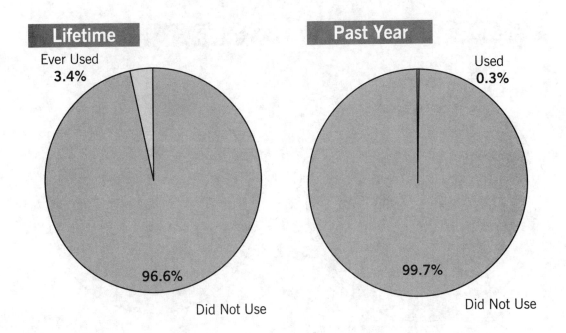

Lifetime

Ever Used
3.4%

96.6%

Did Not Use

Past Year

Used
0.3%

99.7%

Did Not Use

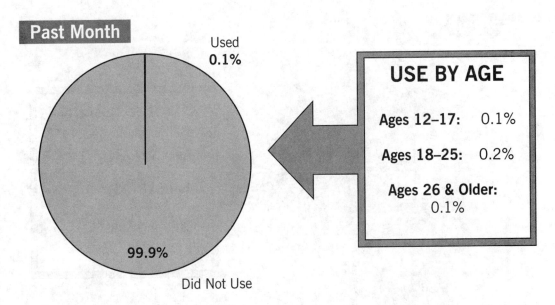

Past Month

Used
0.1%

99.9%

Did Not Use

USE BY AGE

Ages 12–17: 0.1%

Ages 18–25: 0.2%

Ages 26 & Older: 0.1%

* 2007 National Survey on Drug Use & Health

Nonmedical Stimulant Use by Persons
12 Years and Older in the United States*

Where Do You Fit In?

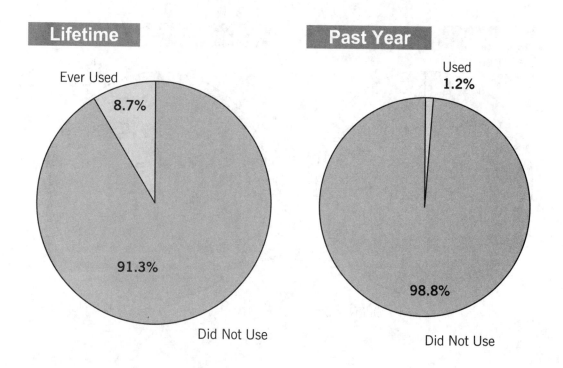

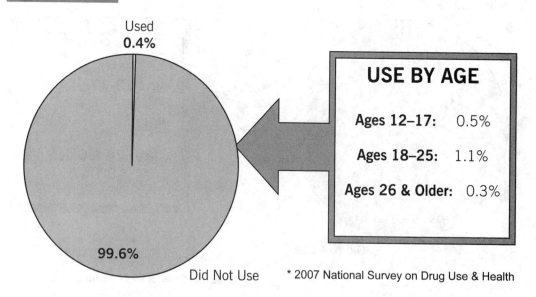

* 2007 National Survey on Drug Use & Health

Nonmedical Tranquilizer Use by Persons
12 Years and Older in the United States*

Where Do You Fit In?

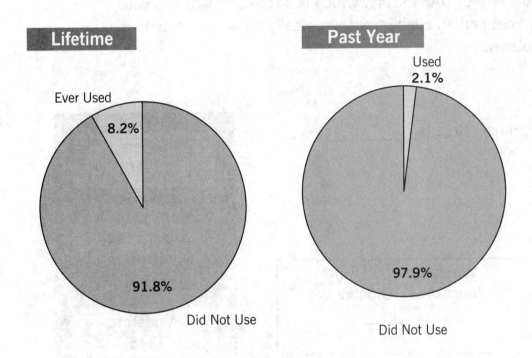

Lifetime

Ever Used
8.2%

91.8%

Did Not Use

Past Year

Used
2.1%

97.9%

Did Not Use

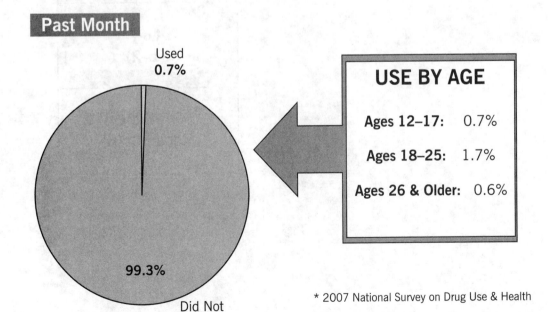

Past Month

Used
0.7%

99.3%

Did Not
Use

USE BY AGE

Ages 12–17: 0.7%

Ages 18–25: 1.7%

Ages 26 & Older: 0.6%

* 2007 National Survey on Drug Use & Health

v

Where Does Your DRUG Use Fit In?

The DAST-10 score evaluates the level of a person's drug problem. Below is your DAST score, which is based on materials you filled out earlier. Higher scores typically reflect more serious problems.

My primary drug is_____

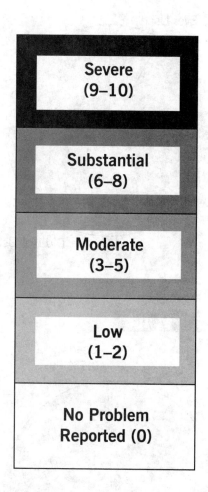

Severe
(9–10)

Substantial
(6–8)

Moderate
(3–5)

Low
(1–2)

No Problem
Reported (0)

Where Do You Fit In?
Your DAST-10 Score is

_____

Example of Personalized Alcohol Use Feedback
Pretreatment to Session 4
Individual and Group Session 4

Personalized feeback for _____

The information you provided about your drinking when you first came in and over the course of treatment is shown in the graphs below.

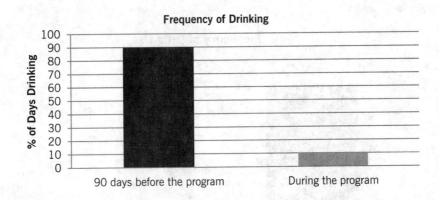

The first graph compares how frequently (% of days) you drank during the 90 days preceding your treatment and during the time you were in the program.

In looking at this first graph, how would you say your drinking has changed?

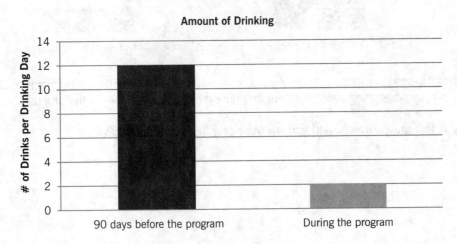

The second graph compares how much you drank per drinking day during the 90 days preceding your treatment and during the time you were in the program.

In looking at this second graph, how would you say your drinking has changed?

Example of Personalized Drug Use Feedback
Pretreatment to Session 4
Individual and Group Session 4

Personalized feeback for _____

Primary drug for which you sought treatment _____

Information you provided about your drug use when you first came in and over the course of treatment is shown in the graph below.

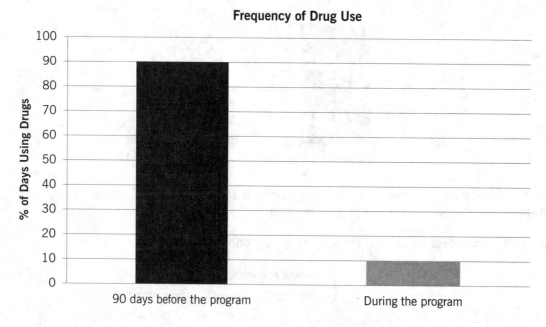

Frequency of Drug Use

(y-axis: % of Days Using Drugs, scale 0 to 100)

90 days before the program   During the program

This graph compares how frequently (% of days) you used the drug for which you sought treatment during the 90 days preceding your treatment and during the time you were in the program.

In looking at this graph, how would you say your drug use has changed?

Reading on Identifying Triggers
Individual and Group Session 2

- Problems don't usually develop overnight, and they usually don't disappear overnight.
- For some people, it may be smooth sailing from the day they decide to change, but for others change takes time.
- Think about changing as an attempt to climb a mountain. Some people are able to climb Mt. Change quickly via Trail B. For others, this climb, as shown in the diagram below via Trail A, may take time.
- While most people make steady progress, some will hit dips in the trail that can slow them down, but that doesn't have to stop them. For example, if you are on a diet and go off it for one day, you can view this in one of two ways.
  1. As a **failure**, give up, and return to your old eating patterns. Doing this will not help you reach your goal.
  2. As a **temporary setback.** By doing this you have a better chance of achieving your goal.

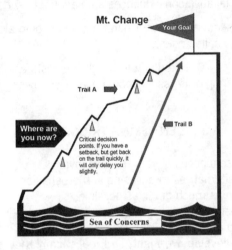

UNDERSTANDING THE PROBLEM

Although we sometimes do things that are not good for us, there are usually reasons why we behave in certain ways. The first step in trying to change a behavior is to identify why it occurs.

TRIGGERS

Triggers are things that often lead to problem behaviors. Many circumstances can act as triggers, such as pleasant or unpleasant emotions or just routine situations. For example:

- **Unexpected situations:** Your plane is delayed; the job you were expecting falls through.
- **Situations you seek:** Going to a party.

(cont.)

- **Emotional situations (positive or negative):** An argument; bumping into an old friend; being bored; celebrating.
- **Stressful personal situations:** Financial problems; a job interview; court appearance.

As you can see, trigger situations can vary greatly. Sometimes it may be a single trigger, whereas at other times it may be several triggers.

CONSEQUENCES

If people get an immediate payoff from doing something, they will tend to do it again. **Positive consequences** can include a change in mood, feeling more comfortable with others, or having a good time.

Unfortunately, some behaviors can produce **negative consequences,** such as health problems, family conflicts, or arrests. Although negative consequences are serious, they don't always occur immediately.

When you think about the consequences of your behavior, you should also consider things that could develop in the future. These are called **risks.**

In the decisional balance exercise, we asked you to weigh the costs and benefits of changing. The next step is to identify what is triggering or is associated with your behavior.

IDENTIFYING TRIGGERS

- Identify the triggers and consequences of your risky behavior.
- Develop options or realistic alternatives to engaging in the behavior.
- State your options as goals in as much detail as possible.
- Decide which options are best for you.
- Next, develop action plans to accomplish your goals. Allow a reasonable time period to achieve your goals. **Your problems didn't develop overnight, and realistically they may not disappear overnight.**
- Monitor your progress. If your plan works, take the credit you deserve. If it isn't working, find out why and look for other options.

Example: Identifying Triggers and Consequences
Briefly describe one of your **most serious** risky or problem situations.   Going to a party when stressed.
Describe as specifically as possible the types of **triggers** usually associated with this situation.   Unwinding after work, social pressure, having a few drinks with friends
Describe the **consequences** usually associated with this situation. Remember to consider **negative** and **positive** consequences.   **Positive:** felt good, relaxed   **Negative:** tired in the morning, missed work

(cont.)

136

EXAMPLE: OPTIONS
Problem or Risky Behavior Going to a party when stressed.
Options and Consequences: Describe at least two options and their likely consequences for this problem or risky behavior.
Option 1: Avoid going to the party. **Likely Consequence of Option 1:** **Positive:** Will not drink. **Negative:** Will feel like I'm missing my friends.
Option 2: Going to the party, but limit my drinking to two beers. **Likely Consequence of Option 2:** **Positive:** Able to enjoy friends. **Negative:** May be difficult initially.

EXAMPLE: ACTION PLAN
For each option, develop an action plan that would help you achieve that option.
Best Option: Go to the party and limit my drinking. **Action Plan:** Have a soda between drinks. Pour your own drinks. After two drinks, only have soft drinks. Have something to eat. Make a commitment to leave at a certain time. Enlist a friend to help.
Second Best Option: Don't go to the party. **Action Plan:** Go somewhere that's rewarding like a movie, dinner, or a sporting event with friends.

Exercise on Identifying Triggers
Individual and Group Session 2

Part of this program involves completing readings and homework exercises prior to your sessions. These are intended to help you

- Prepare for your sessions
- Take an active role in changing your behavior
- Evaluate your progress

In the first exercise you weighed the costs and benefits of changing. Now we want to help you identify what is triggering or associated with the behavior you want to change.

THINGS TO CONSIDER WHEN COMPLETING THIS EXERCISE

Because the behavior you want to change has come to play a major or large role in your life, you may need to make some lifestyle changes. Take a look at the following areas in your life:

- **Availability**: If the things that prompt your behavior are readily available, you may want to change your environment.
- **Activities:** If you spend a lot of time engaging in the behavior, you may need to find other ways to spend your time.
- **Relationships with peers**: In some cases, a change in social relationships may be necessary to change behaviors. If you decide that associating with certain people is too risky, then you might decide that a change in your circle of friends is necessary.

The following questions and general categories of triggers are intended to help you complete this exercise.

Questions:

- Where and when does your behavior occur?
- What other people are present on these occasions and how do they affect your behavior?
- What do you accomplish by engaging in the behavior? That is, what purpose does it serve for you?

General Categories of Triggers:

- **Emotional State** (e.g., angry, depressed, happy, sad)
- **Physical State** (e.g., relaxed, tense, tired, aroused)
- **Presence of Others** (e.g., when the behavior occurs are certain people present?)
- **Availability**
- **Physical Setting** (e.g., work, party, ex-spouse's house)
- **Social Pressure** (e.g., are you forced or coerced into doing things you don't want to?)
- **Activities** (e.g., work, working at home, playing sports, watching TV, playing cards)
- **Thoughts** (e.g., remember times you engaged in the behavior)

You are now ready to complete this exercise!

(cont.)

EXERCISE

Describe **two general types of situations** that have triggered the behavior you want to change.

One thing that can help you to identify triggers and consequences related to changing is to think about real experiences you have had.

TRIGGER SITUATION 1

Briefly describe **ONE** of your **high-risk trigger situations**.

_____

_____

_____

_____

_____

_____

_____

_____

Describe the types of **CONSEQUENCES** usually associated with this situation. Consider both **NEGATIVE** and **POSITIVE** consequences, and whether they occur right away or are delayed.

_____

_____

_____

_____

_____

_____

_____

_____

(cont.)

TRIGGER SITUATION 2

Briefly describe **ONE** of your **high-risk trigger situations**.

_____

_____

_____

_____

_____

_____

_____

_____

_____

Describe the types of **CONSEQUENCES** usually associated with this situation.
Consider both **NEGATIVE** and **POSITIVE** consequences, and whether they occur
right away or are delayed.

_____

_____

_____

_____

_____

_____

_____

_____

_____

_____

Sample BSCQ Alcohol or Drug Use Profile from the Assessment
Individual and Group Session 2

YOUR SELF-CONFIDENCE PROFILE

The following graph shows your confidence that you could resist drinking heavily or resist urges to use drugs in different situations. Situations in which you have low confidence are more likely to pose a risk for you. You may find it particularly helpful to think of ways to identify and plan for these situations in advance. For example, if you have little confidence that you can resist drinking heavily or using drugs in social pressure situations, you may want to avoid such situations or deal with them differently. You can also look at your daily alcohol or drug use calendar to see if your heavier drinking days or drug use occurred when you had trouble resisting urges to drink heavily or resisting urges to use drugs.

How Confident Are You?

The three situations in which you indicated you had the lowest confidence in your ability to resist drinking heavily or resist using drugs are highlighted in **BLACK** below.

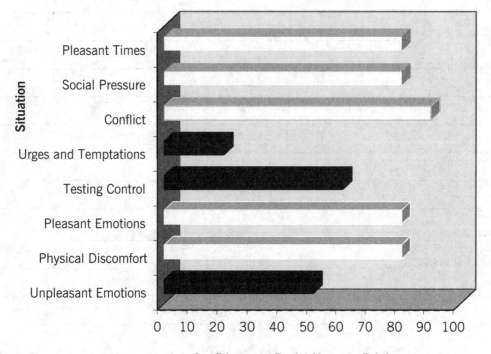

**Confidence to Resist Urges to Drink
Heavily or Resist Urges to Use Drugs**

Exercise on Developing New Options and Plans
Individual and Group Session 3

In this exercise you will develop new options and action plans for the high-risk trigger situations you described in the exercise on **Identifying Triggers**.

TRIGGER SITUATION 1

Describe two options and their likely consequences for your **first trigger situation** in the exercise on **Identifying Triggers**.

- Be as **specific** as possible in describing your options, all of which should be **feasible**.
- **For each option**, describe what you think would happen if you used that option.
- Consider **both negative and positive** consequences.
- Finally, **decide which option** would be your best and second-best option for dealing with this trigger situation.

- **Option 1:** _____

Likely Consequences: _____

_____

_____

_____

_____

_____

_____

- **Option 2:** _____

Likely Consequences: _____

_____

_____

_____

_____

_____

_____

(cont.)

CHANGE PLAN

You have selected two options for your Trigger Situation 1. **For each option**, describe what you need to do to achieve that option.

- Your **Change Plan** should describe in some detail **how you could put your option into practice**.
- It helps to break your plan into **smaller steps**.

- **Option # 1 Change Plan**

_____

_____

_____

_____

_____

_____

_____

_____

- **Option # 2 Change Plan**

_____

_____

_____

_____

_____

_____

_____

_____

_____

(cont.)

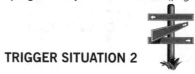

TRIGGER SITUATION 2

Describe two options and their likely consequences for your **second trigger situation** in the exercise on **Identifying Triggers**.

- Be as **specific** as possible in describing your options, all of which should be **feasible**.
- **For each option**, describe what you think would happen if you used that option.
- Consider **both negative and positive** consequences.
- Finally, **decide which option** would be your best and second-best option for dealing with this trigger situation.

- **Option 1:** _____

Likely Consequences: _____

_____

_____

_____

_____

_____

_____

- **Option 2:** _____

Likely Consequences: _____

_____

_____

_____

_____

_____

_____

(cont.)

CHANGE PLAN

You have selected two options for your Trigger Situation 1. **For each option**, describe what you need to do to achieve that option.

- Your **Change Plan** should describe in some detail **how you could put your option into practice**.
- It helps to break your plan into **smaller steps**.

- **Option # 1 Change Plan**

_____
_____
_____
_____
_____
_____
_____
_____
_____

- **Option # 2 Change Plan**

_____
_____
_____
_____
_____
_____
_____
_____
_____

Sample BSCQ Alcohol or Drug Use Profile
from the Assessment and Session 3
Individual and Group Session 4

YOUR SELF-CONFIDENCE PROFILE

How Confident Are You?

The following graph shows your confidence that you could resist drinking heavily or resist urges to use drugs in different situations. The **GRAY** bars show your confidence when you started the program and the **BLACK** bars show how confident you are now. Situations in which you have low confidence are more likely to pose a risk for you. Remember, you may need to avoid situations in which you still have low confidence that you can resist drinking heavily or resist urges to use drugs, or learn to deal with them differently.

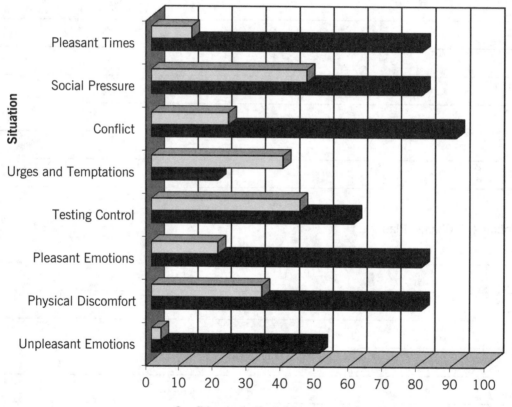

**Confidence to Resist Urges to Drink Heavily
or Resist Urges to Use Drugs**

Request for Additional Sessions
Individual and Group Session 4

- This treatment program allows you to request additional individual sessions beyond the first four sessions.

- The program is designed to be individualized. Some people will need more sessions than others; some may need more now, some may need more later.

- Consistent with being a program that allows each individual to guide his or her own change, if you feel you require additional sessions, you need only to ask your therapist.

- In addition, your therapist will be contacting you by phone one month after your last session. This contact allows your therapist to find out how you are doing and also allows you an opportunity to discuss any issues or problems you are concerned about or request additional sessions.

- Please check the option below that reflects what you feel you need at the present time and give this form to your therapist at the beginning of your next session.

    a. _____ I do not feel I need any further sessions beyond the next session, but I understand I can call and request additional sessions at any time in the future.

    b. _____ I feel I need _____ additional sessions at this time, for the following reasons:

    _____

    _____

    c. _____ I would like to discuss the issue of whether I need additional sessions with my therapist at the next treatment session.

CHAPTER 5

Integrating Motivational Interviewing and Cognitive-Behavioral Techniques into Group Therapy

Although some CBT [cognitive-behavioral therapy] groups do currently employ group processes, little attention had been focused on how a CBT group can systematically use group power to maximize efficacy or how CBT interventions might impact upon group process.
—SATTERFIELD (1994, p. 185)

A **pure motivational interviewing psychotherapy group** [original emphasis] could be developed in which a skillful counselor utilized motivational interviewing techniques and adhered to motivational interviewing principles within the group.
—INGERSOLL, WAGNER, AND GHARIB (2002, p. 52)

This chapter discusses issues concerning difficulties that others have encountered when attempting to extend cognitive-behavioral and motivational interviewing methods to a group therapy context. It also includes a brief review of the few RCTs that have been conducted comparing individual and group treatments for SUDs.

Motivational interviewing is designed to develop a collaborative relationship between clients and therapists in which clients' resistance is minimized and their commitment to change is strengthened and sustained. In addition to treating SUDs, studies using motivational interviewing have had impressive outcomes across a variety of health and mental health problems (Britt et al., 2003; Burke et al., 2003; Heather, 2005; Miller, 2005; Resnicow et al., 2002; Wright, 2004). However, most studies have only involved treatment delivered in an individual setting. The successful adaptation of motivational interviewing to group therapy, in contrast, has been difficult (Walters, Bennett, & Miller, 2000; Walters, Ogle, & Martin, 2002). In their review of motivational interviewing in groups, Walters and colleagues (2002) found that when motivational interviewing was used in the context of providing psychoeducational feedback to participants in groups it was not successful. Often this involved a single session done in a non–motivational interviewing manner to correct deficient knowledge. In many ways, such psychoeducational efforts are better characterized as lecturing or as conducting individual therapy in a group setting compared with group psychotherapy that utilizes group processes to facilitate behavior change.

In their review of failed group motivational interviewing studies, Walters and colleagues (2000) may have inadvertently provided an explanation for the limited success of motivational interviewing group studies:

> Unlike patient education, motivational interviewing is more a navigation process than a transmission of information: Behavior change happens when the individual weighs relevant reasons in relation to the short-term rewards of the behavior. Because of the complexity of interactions in a group, there is more potential for discrepancy diffusion, non-participation, resistance, and collective argumentation. (p. 381)

Another way of understanding why motivational interviewing does not adapt particularly well to psychoeducational and many support groups is to realize that although "the group is a vehicle for delivering a particular package of theoretical material, the nature of the member interaction is not the prime focus" (MacKenzie, 1994, pp. 47–48). In traditional group psychotherapy, MacKenzie (1994) says that the members' interactional experience is the primary learning vehicle. In a related regard, Ingersoll and her colleagues (2002), in recognizing that their motivational group model was psychoeducational in nature, stated that "A *pure motivational interviewing psychotherapy group* could be developed in which a skillful counselor utilized motivational interviewing techniques and adhered to motivational interviewing principles within the group" (p. 52, original emphasis).

THE POWER OF THE GROUP: CAPITALIZING ON GROUP PROCESSES

Almost all cognitive-behavioral treatments are evidence-based and have been shown to be effective with a host of clinical disorders in an individual setting (see Bieling, McCabe, & Antony, 2006; Satterfield, 1994). Although cognitive-behavioral therapies have traditionally been conducted in an individual format, an increasing number of studies have extended these treatments to a group setting. Despite this expansion, as discussed shortly, RCTs comparing group and individual treatments, particularly the same treatment, have been few in number (Tucker & Oei, 2007). Two reviews, published over a decade apart, have compared cognitive-behavioral therapy in group versus individual settings and both reviews concluded that the results were mixed or inconsistent (Satterfield, 1994; Tucker & Oei, 2007). Satterfield (1994) suggested that many group cognitive-behavioral treatment studies have "deemphasized group dynamics" (p. 187).

Two major problems that have plagued cognitive-behavioral group treatments are (1) their failure to systematically use group processes, which Satterfield (1994) says "dilutes their power" (p. 192), and (2) their failure to integrate cognitive-behavioral techniques with group processes. These concerns, articulated 15 years ago (Satterfield, 1994), were reiterated recently in a book on this topic (Bieling et al., 2006). In his 1994 review, Satterfield argued that most cognitive-behavioral therapy groups seemed to view group dynamics as "epiphenomenal or minimize the importance of group processes to varying degrees" (p. 185), and, "although interpersonal exchanges do occur in CBT [cognitive-behavioral therapy] groups, interventions usually focus on treating the individual in a group rather than through the group" (Satterfield, 1994, p. 185). In addition, both Satterfield and Bieling and colleagues have asserted that when cognitive-behavioral groups target the intervention to individuals in the group, they ignore the power of the group.

For example, in a behavioral study involving social skills training groups, Monti and colleagues (1989) reported that their groups were intended "to educate clients rather than explore feelings" (p. 126). They further commented, "in the context of behavioral skills training groups, 'process' can have a somewhat different meaning than it does when it is used in more traditional group psychotherapy" (p. 125). Similarly, in describing how to deliver cognitive-behavioral treatment for social phobia in a group setting, Heimberg and Becker (2002) cautioned that in terms of their group instruction many of the activities "focus on the interaction of the therapist(s) with a single client" (p. 268). As with Monti and colleagues' study, Heimberg and Becker's skills training groups for social phobia can be viewed as dyadic interactions conducted in a group context rather than as reflecting true group processes. In summary, cognitive-behavioral studies typically have been highly structured, and they often have involved a therapist working with one client at a time while other group members observe the interaction. This, of course, is very different from using interactions among group members as a force for change.

Satterfield (1994) suggested that attention to group processes and structure could enhance the outcomes of cognitive-behavioral therapy studies. In looking at some of the key group process variables identified by Satterfield (e.g., group cohesion, group norms, isomorphism), it is easy to understand why successful cognitive-behavioral interventions and motivational interviewing techniques conducted in an individual setting have not readily generalized to a group setting. For example, group cohesion, discussed in detail in Chapter 6, is defined as the extent to which a group is reinforcing to its members. Cohesive groups are characterized as having a positive group atmosphere, a culture in which members take personal responsibility for group work and for group changes. Cohesive groups also have an absence of interpersonal tension. Thus groups that fail to use group processes are more likely to have low levels of cohesion, a characteristic that research has found to be associated with poorer treatment outcomes (MacKenzie, 1997; Satterfield, 1994).

A group setting provides a basis for influencing group members' behavior in terms of social support and social pressure to change, something not possible in individual therapy. When group dynamics are operating, interactions are occurring on multiple levels, as well as within the entire group. One reason that group psychotherapy is viewed as complex and challenging is that a therapist has to operate on multiple levels (Dies, 1994; Yalom & Leszcz, 2005): (1) as a member of the group; (2) as a therapist directing the group toward goals and addressing resistive or challenging members; and (3) as discussed in Chapter 6, as an orchestra conductor getting the group members to work in harmony to produce a sound not achievable by any single instrument.

ADAPTATION OF THE GSC TREATMENT MODEL

The preceding chapter described how to conduct GSC treatment using an individual therapy model and contained four individual treatment session outlines for therapists. In contrast, this chapter describes the adaptation of the GSC treatment model to group therapy. This adaptation involves integrating cognitive-behavioral and motivational interviewing strategies and techniques into a group format. As in Chapter 4, at the end of this chapter there are four session handouts for the group leaders (Group Therapist Handouts 5.1–5.4), which describe session objectives, session procedures, client handouts, and pregroup planning. In addition, each group handout presents several round-robin discussions, the format used to conduct the clinical intervention in a therapy group. This discussion format is designed to get support, feedback, and advice emanating primarily from group members rather than the group leaders. Within each round-robin discussion are sample dialogues and clinical examples that allow group leaders to integrate the cognitive-behavioral and motivational interviewing techniques, strategies, and homework exercises into a group format. To avoid redundancy, descriptions of the GSC measures and other session details, explained at length in Chapters 3 and 4, are not repeated here. Rather, reference is made to their having been described in other chapters.

Composition and Structure of the GSC Groups

As described in Chapter 1 (see Table 1.2), several evidence-based studies have evaluated the GSC treatment model. Except for the study described in this book (L. C. Sobell et al., 2009), the other studies were conducted using an individual therapy format. In terms of composition and structure, the GSC group intervention, like its individual counterpart, is a cognitive-behavioral intervention that uses a motivational counseling style and strategies throughout treatment. Because the intervention is time-limited (i.e., assessment and four semistructured sessions), a closed-group format is used (i.e., no members added after the first session).

The client mix can be heterogeneous and include males and females, as well as individuals with different substance abuse problems. The ideal number of members for such groups is six to eight (in addition to the leaders). Group sessions are scheduled once a week for 2 hours. Group members are phoned the day before each meeting to remind them of the upcoming group. Because the GSC group treatment model uses group processes to avoid conducting one-on-one therapy in a group setting, the group leaders (cotherapists) need training in how to use group processes. The same homework exercises, readings, and self-monitoring logs used for conducting individual GSC therapy are used in the group version of the treatment, with the main difference being that the group discussions are conducted using a round-robin discussion format, which is described shortly.

Before starting the group, clients are assessed individually, and the upcoming group is discussed with them. As part of the assessment, they are given a brochure (Client Handout 5.1) that describes the benefits of group therapy and the expectations of group members. Before and after every group, the group leaders meet for 10–15 minutes for pregroup preparation and postgroup discussions. Although there are only four structured sessions, clients can request additional sessions that would be conducted as individual therapy sessions. In our clinical experience, it has worked well for one of the group leaders to be the therapist for members who request further sessions. Finally, all clients are informed that one of the group leaders will call them about 1 month after their last group session to inquire about their progress, to be supportive of changes, and to schedule additional sessions if needed.

Preparing to Lead Groups

As is discussed in Chapters 7 and 8, conducting therapy groups (vs. process or psychoeducational groups) is complex and can present challenges. There are several reasons that group therapy is seen as more complex than individual therapy. The first is that multiple clients must be handled simultaneously. Second, as is discussed in Chapter 9, many group therapists have had little to no formal group training. To meet the challenges of group work and to provide appropriate care for patients, experts in the field of group psychotherapy feel that specialized training is essential (Bieling et al., 2006; Dies, 1994; Markus & King, 2003; Thorn, 2004; Yalom & Leszcz, 2005). Because many of the skills needed to conduct individual therapy do not generalize to group therapy (Dies, 1994), even the best individual therapists will need training to effectively use and apply group processes. Finally, a major reason that it has been difficult to integrate cognitive-behavioral and motivational interventions, especially components such as homework exercises and personalized feedback, into group therapy has been an insufficient appreciation for group processes (Bieling et al., 2006).

Concerns When Adapting Motivational Interviewing and Cognitive-Behavioral Techniques and Strategies into a Group Format

For the reasons just discussed, extending any evidence-based treatment delivered as individual therapy to a group format requires serious adaptations. As discussed in Chapter 1, when we decided to extend the GSC treatment model to a group format, it took considerable planning and work. One of the adaptations involved recognizing the need to understand the dynamics of running groups using group processes. The primary reason for this is that, unlike individual therapy, in which there is a dyadic interaction, in groups there are multiple and complex interactions that need to be managed. A sine qua non of successfully running groups is for group leaders to understand how to use the interactions of the group to guide members toward behavior change (Yalom & Leszcz, 2005) and to "rigorously and responsibly use group processes" (Satterfield, 1994, p. 192).

We had three major concerns when incorporating cognitive-behavioral and motivational interviewing techniques into a group format. The first was ensuring that the treatment would make use of the group format rather than simply being an arena for observing dyadic interactions. In this regard, Satterfield (1994) has asserted that "although interpersonal exchanges do occur in cognitive-behavioral groups, interventions usually focus on treating the individual *in* the group rather than *through* the group" (p. 185, original emphasis). Our second concern was to make sure that group processes were utilized to facilitate change. The third major concern was to integrate motivational and cognitive-behavioral strategies into the group format in a way that would retain their therapeutic impact and effectiveness.

The first two concerns can be addressed if therapists receive adequate training in group processes. In terms of the integration of motivational interviewing and cognitive-behavioral strategies into a group format, which is the main focus of this chapter, we first reviewed the literature on group therapy to learn how to create an effective integration that would capitalize on group processes. We also arranged for experts in group therapy to train the staff. This experience demonstrated to us that therapists with little group experience could be successfully trained in group processes (i.e., outcomes for the group and individual treatment conditions in our study were very similar, and both demonstrated significant pre- to posttreatment changes; L. C. Sobell et al., 2009).

At the same time that we were determining how to integrate cognitive-behavioral and motivational interviewing strategies into a group format, we also had to address constraints inherent in group therapy. The major constraint we faced was including all members in the group discussions within the time limits of the group. In this regard, we decided to use what we have termed round-robin discussions. Thus, for many of the GSC procedures (e.g., personalized feedback, review of homework exercises), the primary way the group sessions differ from the individual sessions is that the groups use a round-robin discussion format.

ROUND-ROBIN DISCUSSIONS

Round-robin discussions are used throughout the GSC group sessions as a way of including all group members in the discussion of all major topics and exercises. Table 5.1 contains descriptions of the several round-robin discussions used in the four GSC group sessions (L. C. Sobell et al., 2009). The four Group Therapist Handouts (5.1–5.4) at the end of this chapter include specific suggestions for how to focus each round-robin discussion and examples of ways the group leaders can initiate and maintain the discussions. In addition, the handouts contain notes for group leaders related to managing the discussions. Table 5.2 provides examples of statements group leaders can make to bring members and topics into the group discussion (e.g., address sensitive issues raised by a member, get all members to comment on a particular topic).

Round-Robin Discussions: A Way for Members to Share Time in Groups

Although group members cannot receive as much attention (e.g., homework answers) as in individual therapy, the round-robin discussions provide an opportunity for all group members to discuss some aspect of each topic or assignment and to receive feedback and support from their peers. At the first session, the following key aspects of group are discussed: expectations of members, group rules, the need for regular participation, and group members' need to act as agents of change (i.e., providing support and reinforcement to one another). Last, for round-robin discussions to work effectively, group leaders need to manage the time so that all members get an opportunity to participate and all topics scheduled for each session are covered (e.g., personalized feedback, discussions of homework).

Group leaders also explain to the group that they are looking for balanced participation and that one way to ensure this is to use round-robin discussions. Although each group member always gets an opportunity to discuss each assignment and his or her weekly self-monitoring logs, each is asked to select one example from the homework (e.g., in Client Handout 4.6, one of the two high-risk trigger situations) rather than discussing everything in each assignment. Over the years, we have found that if the rationale for round-robin discussions is presented to the group, they understand and quickly become accustomed to the procedure.

At every group session, members are asked to share their experiences and to comment on other members' behaviors and assignments. In this way, commonalities among members can be

TABLE 5.1. Round Robin Discussion Topics Used in the GSC Group Treatment

SESSION 1

- *Introductions:* Includes normalizing members' feelings about groups and discussing group rules, what members expect out of treatment, and why they come to treatment
- *Self-Monitoring Logs:* Discussion of clients' completed logs for alcohol or drug use since the assessment interview (Alcohol: Client Handout 3.2; Drug: Client Handout 3.3)
- *Goal Evaluations:* Review of clients' completed goal evaluations for abstinence or low-risk, limited drinking, including their goal importance and confidence ratings (Abstinence: Client Handout 3.4; Goal Choice: Client Handout 3.5)
- *Personalized Feedback:* Discussion of the personalized feedback handouts (i.e., summaries of pretreatment alcohol and drug use; where their alcohol or drug use fits in with respect to national norms; scores on the AUDIT or DAST-10 evaluating the seriousness of their pretreatment substance use (Alcohol: Client Handout 4.1; Drug: Client Handout 4.2).
- *Decisional Balance:* Discussion of good and less good things about changing alcohol or drug use using the decisional balance exercise (Client Handout 3.1)
- *End of Session:* Wrap-Up and what stood out

SESSION 2

- *Self-Monitoring Logs:* Discussion of clients' completed logs for alcohol or drug use since Session 1 (Alcohol: Client Handout 3.2; Drug: Client Handout 3.3)
- *High-Risk Trigger Situations:* Discussion of the reading and exercise on identification of high-risk trigger situations for alcohol and drug use, including how to take a realistic perspective on change (i.e., Mt. Recovery) and how to view slips as learning experiences (Reading: Client Handout 4.5; Exercise: Client Handout 4.6)
- *BSCQ:* Review of the personalized profiles of high-risk situations for alcohol or drug use using the BSCQ clients completed at assessment; includes a discussion of the relationship of the BSCQ profile to their high-risk triggers homework exercise (Client Handout 4.7)
- *Where Are You Now Scale:* Review of clients' completed Where Are You Now scale (Client Handout 3.6)
- *End of Session:* Wrap-Up and what stood out

SESSION 3

- *Self-Monitoring Logs:* Discussion of clients' completed logs for alcohol or drug use since Session 2 (Alcohol: Client Handout 3.2; Drug: Client Handout 3.3)
- *Developing New Options and Action Plans:* Discussion of the homework exercise on developing new options and action plans to deal with the high-risk trigger situations identified in Session 2 (Client Handout 4.8)
- *End of Session:* Wrap-Up and what stood out

SESSION 4

- *Self-Monitoring Logs:* Discussion of clients' completed logs for alcohol or drug use since Session 3 (Alcohol: Client Handout 3.2; Drug: Client Handout 3.3)
- *Personalized Comparative Feedback about Alcohol or Drug Changes:* Discussion of personalized feedback about changes in alcohol or drug use from the assessment session through Session 3 (Client Handouts 4.3 and 4.4, respectively)
- *Comparative Goal Evaluations:* Comparative evaluation of clients' first (assessment) and second (Session 3) goal evaluations, including their goal importance and confidence ratings (Abstinence: Client Handout 3.4; Goal Choice: Client Handout 3.5)
- *Revisiting the Decisional Balance Exercise:* Discussion of any additions or changes in clients' decisional balance exercise answers from Session 1 through Session 4
- *BSCQ Changes:* Review of the prepared personalized profiles of clients' high-risk situations for alcohol or drug use using the BSCQ completed at assessment and at Session 3 (Client Handout 4.9)
- *Implementation of Options:* Discussion of implementation of the exercise relating to new options to deal with the high-risk trigger situations
- *Revisiting Mt. Recovery and Relapse Prevention:* Review of the high-risk triggers reading
- *Where Are You Now Scale:* Comparative review of the clients' completed Where Are You Now scale (Client Handout 3.6) over treatment
- *End of Session:* Wrap-Up and what stood out

TABLE 5.2. Ways to Bring Different Members and Topics into Group Discussions

Group focus	Leaders' comments
Look for commonalities in the discussion.	• *"Who else has had that kind of experience?"* • *"Who else has similar feelings?"* • *"Who else feels the same way as Mary?"*
Include more group members in the discussion.	• *"What does the group think are some reasons why someone might decide to drink or use drugs after being abstinent for several months?"*
Invite all members to comment (used with homework exercises).	• *"What stood out about the decisional balance exercise that each of you completed for this session?"*
Elicit supportive statements from the group about other members' changes.	• *"It sounds like several members have made big changes in their substance use since last week. How does the group feel about these changes?"*
Address an issue raised by one member and invite others to comment.	• *"It sounds like Bill is ambivalent about not using cocaine. How have others dealt with similar feelings?"*
Get other members to provide additional suggestions.	• *"Okay, so Bill has provided one suggestion for how Mary might handle her difficulties with her daughter. What other options can the group think of to help Mary?"*
Get all members to comment on a particular topic.	• *"How would each of your lives be different six months from now if you stopped using alcohol and drugs?"*
Invite others to provide alternative responses to one member's harsh response.	• *"Mary, that is one way of looking at what has happened to Bill. What are some other ways of looking at what happened with Bill?"*
Address an uncomfortable interaction and invite others to comment.	• *"I am getting the sense that others seem to be uncomfortable with what has just happened."*
Address tension that has arisen between group members; group leaders call a time-out to process what has happened.	• *"It sounds like a lot is happening, and I want to call a 'time-out.' We can come back to the topic later, but let's look at what is happening in the group right now."*
Address a sensitive issue raised by a member and invite others to comment.	• *"Mary has revealed some very personal things about herself. That must have been difficult. How do others in the group feel about what Mary just shared?"*
Acknowledge members' nonverbal responses and invite them to translate nonverbal responses into verbal responses.	• *"I noticed when Mary discussed her difficulties with her husband, that many of you were nodding in agreement. What do the head nods mean?"*

identified and group members are given an opportunity to provide support for or critiques of other members' behaviors. Except for structured group activities (e.g., homework assignments), it is not necessary to have all members participate in every round-robin discussion. All members should, however, participate in each group session. What builds group cohesion is not the amount of time that a member participates but, rather, getting everyone actively participating.

Round-robin discussions begin with the group leaders introducing a topic and then opening up the discussion to the group members. If no one initially comments, the group leaders can ask the entire group who would like to start the discussion, or the leaders can ask a specific member to start. When members voluntarily comment in the first few sessions, group leaders should reinforce their comments (e.g., *"This is exactly what we are looking to have members do in group"*).

Round-Robin Discussions and Group Cohesion

Round-robin discussions not only ensure that all group members participate regularly, but they also promote the development of cohesion using group processes (e.g., members identify commonalities and provide supportive comments to other members). To use the group time efficiently during pregroup preparation (see Chapter 6), group leaders need to allocate time to cover the planned session procedures (e.g., Session 1: beginning and ending groups; reviewing self-monitoring logs; discussing members' decisional balance exercises; presenting members with feedback materials; explaining homework exercises for the next session).

A major goal of group therapy is to have the group members, rather than the group leaders, be the main source of reinforcement and support for other members. Besides providing emotional support to each other, group members can also offer one another consensual validation and advice on how to handle problems. As is discussed in the next chapter, the goal is to have the *music come from the group*. Viewed this way, group members should be doing most of the talking, while the group leaders orchestrate the discussions and bring members into the conversations. Early in the formation of the group, the leaders need to encourage participation by all members. Identifying commonalities among members is a key way to develop group cohesion.

Starting and Ending Groups Using Round-Robin Discussions

Because some group members report initial anxiety about speaking in groups, a goal in the first session is to develop a safe climate for sharing and self-disclosure. One way to facilitate this is to start the first group session by having all members introduce themselves. The first session contains several nonthreatening round-robin discussion topics (see the Group Therapist Handout 5.1; e.g., introductions of members, normalizing members' concerns about groups, what members expect out of treatment). Using nonthreatening group discussions during the first part of Session 1 can help establish group cohesion, something that is essential for positive group therapy outcomes (Dies, 1993; Satterfield, 1994; Yalom & Leszcz, 2005).Similarly, in ending group sessions, it is important to do so in a way that maintains cohesion and positive feelings about group therapy. The following shows some ways for group leaders to end groups using round-robin discussions.

USING ROUND-ROBIN DISCUSSIONS TO END GROUPS

- *"What was it like being in your first group session?"* or *"What was it like to hear from others with similar problems?"*

- To promote skill-based acquisitions from session to session, group leaders can ask, *"What can you take away from today's group that you could implement between now and the next group?"*

This next question, which is asked during the last 5 minutes of open and closed groups, in many ways is like a motivational interviewing summary of each member's perspective, including the group leaders, about what happened in the group.

"We have talked about a lot of things in group today. Let's go around and have everyone, including the group leaders, tell us one thing that stood out about the group."

INTEGRATING MOTIVATIONAL INTERVIEWING STRATEGIES AND TECHNIQUES INTO A GROUP FORMAT USING ROUND-ROBIN DISCUSSIONS

This part of the chapter provides specific suggestions about how to use specific motivational interviewing strategies and techniques in a group format using round-robin discussions. Because motivational interviewing strategies were discussed in detail in Chapter 2, only brief descriptions of the techniques as related to their use in round-robin discussions are presented here.

Using Round-Robin Discussions with Homework

Because groups have multiple members, it is not possible to have everyone discuss answers to their homework exercise, as would occur in an individual therapy session. As discussed in Chapter 3, homework has been a mainstay of cognitive-behavioral interventions for many years and has several benefits: (1) it strengthens what is discussed in therapy; (2) members are engaged in treatment outside of sessions; (3) it allows group leaders to point out commonalities during a discussion, which, in turn, provides a basis for building cohesion; (4) written homework exercises help to keep all group members on the same page; and (5) importantly, research has shown that those who comply with homework have better treatment outcomes, perhaps because they are working outside of sessions (Burns & Spangler, 2000; Kazantzis et al., 2000).

A way to avoid or minimize compliance problems with homework is to explain its rationale and how fits into the treatment (Addis & Jacobson, 2000; Kazantzis, Deane, Ronan, & L'Abate, 2005). Discussing the need to complete homework exercises is equally important, whether the treatment format is individual or group. As discussed in Chapter 1, 90% of group clients in the GRIN study (L. C. Sobell et al., 2009) completed and brought their homework and self-monitoring logs to sessions. We believe this high compliance rate is directly related to our therapists' explaining the rationale and importance of doing homework exercises.

The discussion of homework exercises, which involves all group members, starts with the group leaders asking members to discuss what they got out of the homework exercise. The leaders can then ask, *"Who else has had similar experiences?"* Questions like this can be used to identify commonalities among members.

The Identifying Triggers exercise (Client Handout 4.6) provides a good example of how to use homework exercises in a round-robin discussion. This homework exercise, which is handed out and explained to members in Session 1, is discussed with clients in Session 2. This exercise asks clients to identify and discuss two high-risk trigger situations related to their alcohol or drug use that occurred in the preceding year (see Session 2 in Chapter 4). In individual therapy, clients would discuss both trigger situations with their therapists. However, because there is not enough time to have all group members discuss both trigger situations in the group, each member is asked to select and discuss one of their two trigger situations. The trade-off is that although group members have less time to discuss their personal situations, they benefit by sharing their experiences with other group members who can be supportive and who can offer advice about how they have handled similar situations. The Group Therapist Handouts contain discussions of how to present the homework exercises using a round-robin format.

Incomplete Homework

If clients come to group without their homework or self-monitoring logs, we recommend that the group leaders ask them to complete them before or at the start of the group. This, of course, requires that the group leaders check that the various assignments have been completed before starting the group. Although this might seem disruptive, the alternatives (i.e., not having the assignments completed, leaders not knowing whether members have completed their homework) can diminish members' participation.

It is important for group leaders to address noncompliance with homework early because if one or more clients repeatedly do not complete their homework, other members might get the impression that it is not important to do so. However, as discussed earlier, if the group leaders explain the rationale and importance of doing homework at the first session, compliance is usually not a problem. If a group member repeatedly fails to complete the assignments, the group leaders should address this in a nonjudgmental, motivationally enhancing manner (e.g., *"It looks like some folks are struggling to complete their homework before group. I know we are all busy, but I'm wondering what advice others have for how to fit these assignments into one's schedule?"*).

Using Round-Robin Discussions with Personalized Feedback Materials

Groups provide a rich forum for discussing feedback materials. Using round-robin discussions, we have group members comment on the personalized feedback materials we provide them in group. Members are also encouraged to discuss their reactions to the materials. As shown in Table 4.1, several types of motivational feedback handouts are part of the GSC group intervention. The four Group Therapist Handouts contain examples of ways group leaders can present feedback throughout the group sessions. The following example is a generic way of presenting feedback.

> *"We will be giving everyone a lot of information today. The first type of feedback is based on the information you provided in your assessment session and relates to your past alcohol or drug use. The reason we give you feedback about your* [insert risky problem behavior here] *is to provide you with information that you can use to make more informed choices about changing. Let's have everyone look at the personalized graphs we prepared of your* [insert risky problem behavior here] *and tell the group what stands out for you about these summaries."*

Motivation for change often occurs when people recognize a discrepancy in their risky problem behavior (i.e., a difference between how they are acting and how they think they should act). Personalized feedback is one way to address such discrepancies. As discussed in Chapter

2, the way feedback is presented is important. Feedback or information presented in a neutral, nonjudgmental manner is more likely to be positively received by clients than is being lectured to about the negatives of their behavior or told that they have to change. The ultimate objective of providing feedback is for clients to recognize that their risky problem behaviors are not within the norms and, if continued, can result in more serious consequences.

Using Round-Robin Discussions with a Decisional Balance Exercise

The decisional balance exercise (Client Handout 3.1), designed to address ambivalence about changing, asks clients to consider both the good and less good things about changing and not changing their alcohol or drug use (**or other risky problem behaviors**). This exercise is used to help clients recognize that there are rewards associated with their substance use, although those rewards are short term and could result in long-term negative consequences. The discussion of both the good and less good things about engaging in a behavior also helps clients make sense of their actions, and it makes salient that a continuation of the behavior risks highly undesirable outcomes.

As discussed in the first handout for group therapists (5.1), the decisional balance round-robin discussion invites all group members to talk about their responses and what they have learned from this exercise. This discussion provides an excellent opportunity for the group leaders to identify similarities among members and to prompt group discussion about the need to make decisions based on long-term goals. The ultimate objective of a decisional balance exercise is to help clients recognize their ambivalence about changing and to get them thinking about what it would take to change. Although several discussion topics are listed here, all topics do not have to be addressed, only those relevant to the ongoing group discussion.

POSSIBLE DISCUSSION TOPICS FOR USE WITH THE DECISIONAL BALANCE EXERCISE

- *"What did each of you get out of this exercise?"*
- *"How did the use of the decisional balance exercise affect your thinking about your* **[insert risky problem behavior here]***?"*
- *"What are the good and less good things about doing this exercise?"*
- *"What strikes you most about this exercise?"*
- *"What surprised you most about doing this exercise?"*

Using Round-Robin Discussions to Support Self-Efficacy

Group leaders need to recognize small gains that clients make from session to session. Reinforcing gains is best done by getting group members to comment about the positive changes other group members have made. If a group member discusses changes but other members fail to comment, the group leaders need to elicit comments from them by saying something like, *"Bill was drinking thirty drinks per week before he came to group, and now he is down to one or two per day. How does the group feel about what he has done?"* Getting group members to reinforce each others' gains is a good example of how group members serve as agents of change.

Using Round-Robin Discussions to Present Affirmations

An affirmation is a motivational interviewing strategy used to recognize clients' strengths, successes, and efforts to change. Affirmations can be used for individual clients within the group and for the group as a whole. The following are two examples of how to use affirmations in a group:

> *"Everyone has done a good job of completing their decisional balance homework for this week. Now that we have discussed the good things and less good things about each person's substance use, let's go around and see what one thing it would take for each person to change right now."*

> *"When Mary came in she said she could not go a day without using cocaine. As we just heard, she hasn't used for a week. What does that say about her?"*

Using Round-Robin Discussions to Present Reflections and Open-Ended Questions

As in individual therapy, the group leaders can use open-ended questions and reflections to encourage members to contribute to the group. When group leaders use open-ended questions, members' responses are usually richer or tell more of a story (e.g., *"How do people feel about that?"* or *"When you use cocaine, what does it do for you?"*). Open-ended questions can be asked with no particular member in mind, or they can be directed to a specific member if the group leader feels that member can provide relevant comments to another member. The following are some examples of group-focused questions and reflections.

EXAMPLES OF OPEN-ENDED QUESTIONS AND REFLECTIONS FOR GROUP DISCUSSIONS

- *"That sounds like an important issue. Who else can relate to what Bill has said?"*
- *"How does that relate to why each of you is here?"*
- *"How have others handled similar situations?"*
- *"Mary, it sounds like some of your friends have put a lot of pressure on you to drink. How have others dealt with social pressure to drink?"*
- *"Mary, that is one way of looking at how Bill can handle his mother-in-law. What other suggestions can the group give Bill?"*

On occasion, especially when group leaders are concerned about minimal participation by members, questions and reflections can be directed to a particular member rather than the entire group. For example, a group leader might say, *"That sounds like an issue that many can relate to. What about you, Bill?"* At other times, the group leaders might reflect something that is important to a particular member, such as, *"Bill, you appear to be torn about wanting to change."* They might also further explore a topic by saying, *"Mary, can you tell the group about what led to your decision to leave your job?"*

Judicious Reflections Are at the Heart of Group Work

In motivational interviewing, reflections are the primary way of responding to clients. Reflections are important because they validate therapists' understanding of clients' behaviors and they build empathy. When group leaders recognize that a member has said something significant in the group, it is important to have the group (rather than the leaders) focus on what has occurred. For example, the group leader can say, *"Let's spend some time thinking about what Mary has just said."* In this way, the members have the responsibility for interpreting and reflecting the client's comment.

Group Leaders as Process Consultants

Group leaders have the unique role of acting as process consultants. In this regard, their responsibilities include drawing the group's attention to what is important and pointing out appropriate behaviors for the rest of the group. The following are some examples of reflections that group leaders can use for such purposes (see Chapter 2 for additional examples of how to use reflections).

EXAMPLES OF HOW TO USE REFLECTIONS IN GROUP DISCUSSIONS

- *"Mary has just shared some very strong feelings with the group. Let's go around and see how others feel about* [**insert topic related to the discussion**]*."*
- *"It sounds like most members are saying that balancing a career and raising children is very stressful. Let's go around and have those who have had such experiences share how they have handled them and point out what were some of the biggest challenges."*
- *"That sounds like an important issue that Bill has raised. How have others handled similar situations?"*

Group leaders need to reflect group members' responses that are most relevant to the target behavior, and they need to do it in ways that will promote change talk by members. Summary statements, a form of reflections, can also be used to (1) review and highlight relevant information provided by the group, (2) relate a response by one member to an earlier comment by another member, and (3) transition the group discussion from one topic to another.

Using Round-Robin Discussions to Roll with Resistance

Dealing with difficult or resistant clients in individual therapy is usually easier than handling such clients in a group setting. In groups, the problem can be exacerbated if the group leaders attempt to manage a resistant client individually within the group. Suggestions for handling such situations follow. Group cohesion can also be damaged if members with strong personalities monopolize the group or influence other members by discouraging them from talking. Specific ways to handle monopolizing or chatty clients are discussed in Chapter 8. Some disruptions can be avoided by discussing acceptable group behavior (e.g., not talking over other members, not raising voices) at the first group session.

Dealing with Resistance

Group leaders should avoid confronting members in the group. For example, when dealing with an angry group member, the group leaders should pull other members into the conversation and ask how they have dealt with such feelings (e.g., *"Mary, it sounds like you feel you had no choice in coming here and you are angry. If I recall, other group members have had some similar experiences. Who can share with Mary how they have handled such situations?"*). In the end, the group leaders need to summarize what happened in the group (e.g., *"Mary, although you would rather not be in group today, it sounds like the alternative was jail. I think what the group was trying to get you to think about is what alternative seems better for you now?"*).

When dealing with resistant group members, it is important for group leaders to remember two things: (1) "think Group" (Dies, 1994, p. 86) and throw questions and comments back to the group (i.e., pull group members in and ask how others have dealt with such situations and feelings); and (2) group leaders should not interpret any of the group members' comments as a personal attack. The group leader's response (e.g., throwing it back to the group) should be in relation to the leader's role, and not in a personal role.

PREPARING POTENTIAL GROUP MEMBERS DURING THE ASSESSMENT

Prior to the first group meeting, potential group members attend an individual assessment session with a therapist, preferably a therapist who will be one of the group leaders. The assessment procedures have been presented in detail in Chapter 3, but the following procedures should also occur at the end of the assessment for potential group members. All potential group members should be given the "Introduction to Groups" handout (Client Handout 5.1). Providing clients with this handout is not only an essential component of group preparation, but it also represents an opportunity to discuss the value of the group and address any concerns that clients may have about group therapy.

THINGS TO MENTION TO POTENTIAL GROUP MEMBERS AT THE ASSESSMENT

- *"We have a handout about group therapy that addresses some concerns people have had about groups."*

- *"Many studies have found that group treatment works as well as individual treatment."*

- *"Group gives people an opportunity to do several things that they cannot do in individual therapy, such as sharing experiences with other members and learning how others have dealt with similar problems. Group members also receive support from others dealing with similar problems, which in turn allows members to know that they are not alone in trying to change."*

- *"Last, and very importantly, what members share in groups is confidential:* **What is said in group stays in group**!*"*

GROUP THERAPY CAN BE LIMITED BY CULTURAL OR OTHER FACTORS

Although groups can be a highly efficient way to deliver clinical services, there will be some situations in which the applicability of group therapy is limited by cultural or other factors. A specific case we experienced concerns a sister study to the GRIN study that was conducted in Mexico City using GSC materials translated into Spanish. In that study the overwhelming majority of clients were male (Ayala et al., 1997, 1998). Although the individual therapy condition was replicated, it was not possible to replicate the group therapy condition. In fact, not a single group was conducted in the group therapy arm of the study. According to the investigators, this occurred because nearly all of the potential clients were male, and they were not willing to participate in a treatment in which they would be discussing their substance use problems in front of others (which would conflict with the *machismo* aspect of the culture). Thus, although group treatment is cost effective, in Mexico cultural factors prevented implementation of the intervention with male Hispanic/Latino clients.

SUMMARY

The four handouts, 5.1–5.4, for group therapists at the end of this chapter are specifically designed to help group leaders integrate motivational interviewing and cognitive-behavioral strategies and techniques into group therapy, particularly using round-robin discussions. These four group therapist handouts were adapted from the GRIN study protocol (see Sobell & Sobell, 2009). Readers will also find it helpful to refer back to Chapter 4, which describes the GSC treatment components at length.

It is our hope that this chapter, coupled with the description of the treatment model in Chapter 5, describes and illustrates the group adaptation of GSC in sufficient detail to allow therapists to successfully integrate a motivational interviewing approach and cognitive-behavioral techniques to achieve a cohesive therapy group. The remaining chapters further discuss how to conduct effective groups and how to deal with challenges that may arise when conducting group therapy.

Objectives, Procedures, Client Handouts, Pregroup Planning, and Sample Round-Robin Discussions

Group Session 1

INTRODUCTION

Each of the group therapist handouts for group sessions is intended to help group leaders integrate cognitive-behavioral and motivational interviewing techniques and strategies into a group treatment format. Throughout each session, leaders should look for and acknowledge commonalities among members and encourage members to be supportive of other members' changes.

If the group leaders want to keep copies of the group members' homework exercises and self-monitoring logs, they should develop a procedure that allows them to copy the information before or after the group, as members will need the forms during the group.

In each round-robin discussion, there is a list of suggested questions and topics. Although several topics and questions are provided, group leaders need not ask all questions or address all topics; instead, questions and topics should be selected as they relate to what is happening in the group.

SESSION OBJECTIVES

- Review and discuss members' goal evaluations; provide guidelines or information on contraindications for use if appropriate.
- Review members' self-monitoring logs with respect to their goals.
- Provide members with personalized feedback based on assessment measures.
- Evaluate and discuss members' motivation to change.
- Give homework and instructions for Session 2.

SESSION PROCEDURES

- Introduce session, complete any remaining assessment inquiries.
- Review and discuss members' completed self-monitoring logs, copy or record data.
- Give members personalized feedback from assessment forms and discuss.
- Review and discuss members' completed goal evaluation.
- Review and discuss members' completed decisional balance homework answers.
- Ask members the five-million-dollar question; affirm that changing is a "choice" people make.
- End session: What stood out about today's session? Remind members to do homework.

CLIENT HANDOUTS

- Reading: Identifying Triggers (Client Handout 4.5)
- Exercise: Identifying Triggers (Client Handout 4.6)
- Copies of Client Handout 5.1 for the group members when discussing the group rules

(cont.)

PREGROUP PLANNING

Pregroup planning is seen as critical for several reasons: Retention of group members contributes to members' satisfaction, builds group cohesion, and results in positive group outcomes. Although pregroup planning only takes 15 to 20 minutes, it is important to do it prior to every group. Pregroup planning for the first session is more extensive and may take slightly longer than planning for other sessions. It includes the following.

- Review assessment information on all members.
- Know something about each group member before the group starts, including their first names.
  - ◆ Use 3″ × 5″ cards to make brief notes about each member (e.g., age; first name; marital status; problem type, length, and consequences; medical problems; referral reason).
  - ◆ On a separate sheet of paper draw a circular diagram for the group and write in the first names of each member as they sit down at the first session; this allows you to know who is sitting where and to be able to call on clients using their names.
- Arrange the chairs in a circle for the number of expected group members and the two leaders; for better communication, the group leaders' chairs should be positioned opposite one another (to save these chairs place a clipboard or other materials on them ahead of time).
- Have new homework available for members (Client Handouts 4.5 and 4.6).
- Prior to this session prepare and highlight key points in each group member's "Personalized Feedback Handout: Where Does Your Alcohol Use Fit In?" (Client Handout 4.1) or "Where Does Your Drug Use Fit In?" (Client Handout 4.2).

  Note to Group Leaders: To prepare these handouts, use information collected from the TLFB and other measures administered at the assessment and discussed in Chapter 4 (go to *www.nova.edu/ gsc/online_files* for measures and forms).

- Group leaders also need to decide who will take the lead for each of the major discussion topics in this session (e.g., introduction, self-monitoring, homework, ending group).

FIRST ROUND-ROBIN DISCUSSION

- Introduce group leaders and welcome members to group.
- Have members introduce themselves.
- To begin, one of the group leaders can say, *"Why don't we start by spending a few minutes talking about the benefits of group therapy and what groups are about?"*
- In addition to presenting basic information about the group, the leaders can also say, *"Another thing that is important to think about is that each group member is an agent of change, and the goal is to learn from each other and to be supportive of change. Another way of thinking about this is that solutions come from group members, not from the therapists."*
- After this initial discussion, group leaders can say, *"Now that we have gone over the benefits of group and what is expected of group members, what other concerns do group members have?"*
- After going over the basics, the group leader can start by saying, *"Let's go around and have each member tell us what you expect to get out of group."*

Normalize members' feelings about groups by saying, *"Although it's natural for members to initially feel uncomfortable in groups, groups provide members an opportunity to learn from others with similar problems. There are benefits to having members provide advice and feedback to one another."*

(cont.)

Further Discussion Focus: Leaders can ease members into talking in groups with general questions such as, *"Let's go around and have everyone tell us* [**insert one of the following questions here; ask one question one at a time**].*"*

- *"What brought each of you into treatment?"*
- *"Tell us two or three words that best describe you."* Next ask, *"Now, thinking about those words, how do they relate to why you are here?"*

ROUND-ROBIN DISCUSSION

Topic: Group Rules

Because group rules are intended to shape appropriate group behaviors, promote positive group norms, and reduce clients' anxieties, one of the most important discussions that group leaders can have with group members early in the first session relates to group rules. The group rules most commonly advocated and their rationales are listed in Table 5.3. Although every group member should have received a handout describing the group (Client Handout 5.1) at their assessment, each should be given another copy of this handout at the first session.

Each group rule in Table 5.3 needs to be reviewed. They include: maintaining confidentiality, not socializing outside of group, attending group on time and calling if you cannot come to a group, not using alcohol or illicit drugs before group, not discussing absent members in group, completing homework assignments and bringing them to group, participating regularly, and exhibiting appropriate behaviors in groups (i.e., no yelling, no profanity, no use of cell phone during groups, no talking over one another).

ROUND-ROBIN DISCUSSION

Topic: Group Treatment Program

Discussion Focus: Brief review of the GSC treatment program, including mention of the following.

- There will be four 120-minute group sessions, typically with 6 to 10 members.
- Homework exercises and readings will be assigned.
- Members will participate in self-monitoring and goal setting for alcohol or drug use.
- Group members will learn a general approach to problem solving that will help them guide their own change and motivate them to take responsibility for their own change.
- One of the group leaders will call each group member 1 month after the last session to check on how everyone is doing and if more services are needed.

(cont.)

TABLE 5.3. Group Rules and Their Rationales

Confidentiality. Group discussions are confidential: *What is said in group, stays in group!*

> Rationale: Confidentiality is the sine qua non group rule; without it, members are unlikely to share or even come to group.

Do not socialize outside of groups. Although some interactions will occur outside of the group (e.g., waiting room conversations, riding home on public transportation), it is best to avoid having clients socialize with one another while they are in the group.

> Rationale: Socializing outside of the group can undermine clients' treatment by blurring boundary issues. Even if clients go out for coffee after a group, they form a relationship that others cannot share, and the stronger the relationship, the more likely it is to interfere with group interactions.

Attend groups on time. Members are expected to make groups a priority and attend all sessions, arrive on time, and remain for the entire session unless there is an emergency. Members who are unable to attend a session are expected to call beforehand.

> Rationale: Attendance is important, as each meeting builds on the previous session and missed groups cannot be made up.

Do not use alcohol or illicit drugs before group.

> Rationale: Coming to the group under the influence of alcohol or drugs can be disruptive to group interactions and tends to put the focus on the intoxicated member rather than the group as a whole.

Do not talk about group members who are not present.

> Rationale: Members who are not in the group any longer or unable to attend a session cannot speak for themselves. Discussions about absent members can undermine trust in the group.

Complete homework assignments and bring them to group.

> Rationale: Because the completed assignments are discussed in the group, it is disruptive if some members have not completed their assignments. To enhance compliance, therapists need to give members an explanation about the rationale for and the importance of completing assignments (see Chapters 5 and 6).

All members need to participate in all group sessions.

> Rationale: It is important for members to actively participate in the group (i.e., share their problems and feelings with others). Participation is very important, as each member is viewed as an agent of change, helping other members, being supportive, and providing feedback to others.

Exhibit appropriate behaviors in groups. (1) Take turns speaking and do not talk over one another; (2) respect the rights of others to express their opinions; (3) cell phones must be turned off during the group; (4) profanity, screaming, and yelling are not appropriate; strong emotions need to be communicated in a manner that is not disruptive and allows group members to help one another.

> Rationale: Members should be respectful of one another and of the leaders. Individual outbursts or disruptions take the focus off of the group process.

(cont.)

ROUND-ROBIN DISCUSSION

Topic: Review Members' Completed Self-Monitoring Logs for Their Alcohol or Drug Use since the Assessment Interview (Alcohol: Client Handout 3.2; Drug: Client Handout 3.3)

Discussion Focus

- The discussion can start with a group leader saying, *"Let's go over the self-monitoring logs and look at everybody's alcohol and drug use in the past week."* Follow up by asking a member to begin the discussion, *"*[**Insert client name**]*, give us a general picture of what your alcohol or drug use was like this past week?"*
- **Note to Group Leaders:** Unless relevant, avoid specific details of a client's drinking or drug use (i.e., do not have members present a day-by-day description, as this takes too much time and usually is not that informative).
- If major changes have occurred or if a member handled a difficult situation and did not use, the group leaders can ask the group how they feel about the group member's change.

ROUND-ROBIN DISCUSSION

Topic: Goal Evaluations (Abstinence: Client Handout 3.4; Goal Choice: Client Handout 3.5

Note to Group Leaders: When groups have members with both abstinent and low-risk limited drinking goals, the group leaders can start by saying, *"We are going to review each member's goal form and we want you to freely comment on each others' goals and how realistic they are."*

Abstinence Discussion

- Using a motivational interviewing approach, ask group members to discuss reasons for not using alcohol and drugs.
- Group members should provide sound reasons for being abstinent (e.g., relate it to what would be risked by using substances).
- The motivation for abstinence should be, *"I have chosen not to use alcohol or drugs because that is the best way for me to avoid future problems"* rather than trait attributions (i.e., reasons should not be statements such as *"Because I have a disease"* or *"Because I have no will power"*).

Framing abstinence as a choice, albeit a difficult one, allows discussion of how to accomplish change, whereas a statement of inability to change can lead to a self-fulfilling prophecy

Goal Choice Discussion

- This discussion should begin with the leaders explaining that persons with contraindications to drinking are advised not to drink at all and describing the recommended guidelines for those who do not have contraindications and choose a low-risk drinking goal. For any member who has selected a low-risk drinking goal but has contraindications to drinking, the leaders can point out that the member may not have been aware of the contraindication but should now take it into account.
- Ask group members who have selected a low-risk drinking goal and do not have contraindications, *"Have you ever been able to drink at low levels and without problems before?"*

(cont.)

- Group members can also be asked under what conditions low-risk drinking might pose a risk. This discussion can be facilitated by giving members considering a low-risk limited drinking goal a printed set of guidelines that outline risks that can be discussed.

Note to Group Leaders: If a group member's goal exceeds the recommended guidelines or the person wants to engage in low-risk drinking but has contraindications to alcohol use, group leaders should engage other group members to comment on the risks the person would be taking. To prompt other members to comment on those whose goal exceeds the guidelines, ask, *"As we have been listening to everyone describe their goal evaluation, we need to remember that recommended low-risk drinking limits are very low. What advice can group members provide to each other in terms of how realistic other members' goals are?"*

Additional Goal Evaluation Topics: With respect to members' alcohol or drug use goals, group leaders can use the following questions to get group members talking about their goals.

- *"How realistic is your goal?"*
- *"What obstacles, if any, are you experiencing in trying to achieve your goal?"*
- For clients who have made significant changes in their alcohol or drug use, you can ask, *"You made some very major changes in your alcohol or drug use. How were you able to do that and how do you feel about these changes?"*

Members' Goal Evaluations Related to Their Confidence in Achieving Their Goals and the Importance of Their Goals

- Group leaders can open the discussion by saying, *"Now that we have discussed everyone's goal, let us look at the second part of the goal evaluation, where everyone was asked to evaluate the importance and confidence of achieving their goal. To start, let's look at what everyone put down for the importance of their goal and why you chose your rating."*
- During this discussion, the group leaders should look for commonalities. Several members will not rate reaching their goal as the most important thing in their lives, but instead will rate other things (e.g., health, job) as more important. With this discussion, the idea is to encourage members to discuss the importance of changing.
- After a discussion of the importance, the group leaders can move on to how confident members are in achieving their goals by asking, *"Okay, now let's do the same thing for everyone's confidence ratings."*
- Ask group members, *"What number did you put down for how confident you are right now in terms of reaching your goal, and why?"* This could be followed up with, *"What would have to happen for your goal to go from a [**insert current #**] to a [**higher #**]?"*

ROUND-ROBIN DISCUSSION

Topic: Discussion of Personalized Feedback Handouts (i.e., summaries of pretreatment alcohol use, Client Handout 4.2; drug use, Client Handout 4.3)

Note to Group Leaders: Each member's personalized feedback summary should have been prepared in advance and highlighted (e.g., yellow marker) on the printout you will give all group members during this discussion (i.e., highlight aspects of alcohol or drug use you want members to notice).

(cont.)

Discussion Focus: The crucial aspect of the feedback is comparing group members' personal alcohol or drug use with normative data on substance use. Having members comment on their personalized feedback engages them in a discussion about their current substance use and risk as opposed to group leaders telling them such information. The intent is for group leaders to generate discussion so members understand that their present alcohol or drug use is not normative and that if they continue, such use is predictive of long-term risks (i.e., negative consequences).

Feedback Based on the Timeline Followback That Members Completed at the Assessment (Alcohol Use: Client Handout 4.1; Drug Use: Client Handout 4.2)

Start by giving group members their personalized feedback summaries.

- *"If you remember, we asked each of you many questions about your alcohol and drug use at the assessment, and one thing you did was to fill out a calendar describing your alcohol or drug use prior to entering treatment. We will be giving everyone feedback today about your alcohol or drug use so you can use this information to make more informed decisions about changing your alcohol or drug use. Let's have everyone look at the pie charts and tell the group what stands out about these summaries for you."*
- With alcohol clients, it is not unusual for them to be surprised at how heavy their drinking is compared with the general population, especially if many of their friends also drink heavily. Similarly, drug clients also report to us that they are surprised that so very few (e.g., ≤ 1%) people used many of the illicit drugs such as heroin or cocaine in the previous year.

Feedback Based on the AUDIT (Client Handout 4.1) and DAST-10 (Client Handout 4.2)

- *"At the assessment interview, we also asked you about consequences you might have experienced because of your alcohol or drug use over the past year. Your answers yielded a score that reflects the severity of your alcohol (AUDIT) or drug (DAST-10) use. It is on the last page of your feedback summary. Let's look at these graphs and your scores and tell the group what stands out about this feedback."*
- For surprised members, group leaders can say, *"A few of you look surprised at the feedback. What's surprising about it?"*

ROUND-ROBIN DISCUSSION

Topic: Decisional Balance Exercise (Client Handout 3.1)

Discussion Focus: This exercise, a motivational tool designed to help clients understand their ambivalence and why changing might be difficult, involves a discussion of group members' reports of good and less good things about changing their alcohol or drug use. Listing both the short- and long-term costs and benefits in one place can help them justify and strengthen decisions about changing. Throughout this discussion, group members are invited to comment on their perceptions of other members' statements about the good and less good things related to their alcohol and drug use and what it would take to change. Possible group discussion topics include

- *"What did each of you get out of this exercise?"*
- *"How did the use of a decisional balance exercise affect your thinking about your alcohol or drug use?"*

(cont.)

- *"What good and less good things had you not recognized before doing this exercise?"*
- *"What surprised you most about doing this exercise?"*

Note to Group Leaders: Members' discussion about their decisional balance exercises should include some mention of the following.

- What they recognized about their reasons for drinking or using drugs (i.e., good things about use)
- Potential obstacles to change

ROUND-ROBIN DISCUSSION

Topic: Five-Million-Dollar Question (Client Handout 3.1)

Discussion Focus: After discussing members' decisional balance exercises, ask the group, *"What if you were each offered five million dollars to not use alcohol or drugs for just one day? What would you do?"*

Note to Group Leaders: The Five-Million-Dollar Question is used to show members that for a price, they would change their behavior. The important point from this exercise is that, although change might be difficult, it is a choice people can make. This point can often be made after members report why they would change.

Remember to invite group members to comment on each other's responses to the Five-Million-Dollar Question. To make the point that change is possible, group leaders can say, *"Since we do not have five million dollars, what would be your personal price for changing your alcohol or drug use?"* or *"What would it take for each of you to tip the scale in favor of changing?"*

Homework Assignments for Session 2: Identifying Triggers Reading (Client Handout 4.5) and Exercise (Client Handout 4.6)

- Give each group member the Identifying Triggers reading and exercise
- Tell group members, *"This is a short reading and homework exercise to complete for our next group meeting. The exercise is intended to help you identify your high-risk situations for alcohol or drug use and the consequences of use. Usually, the reasons for using are short-term consequences. What we are asking you to do is explained in the handout. When you complete this homework and bring it back to the next group, it provides an opportunity to talk more about these high-risk trigger situations and to examine why they've been a problem for you. A future homework will help you develop ways of handling those situations by doing things other than using alcohol or drugs."*
- *"The reading will help you understand how to complete the homework and also will help you consider taking a long-term perspective on changing your alcohol or drug use. The reading and exercise are easy to complete and should take about 10 minutes."*
- Finally, tell group members that next week you will have them select one of their two high-risk triggers from the exercise to discuss further.

(cont.)

ROUND-ROBIN DISCUSSION

Topic: End of Session 1, Wrap-Up, and What Stood Out

Have each group member and the leaders comment on their group experience and one thing that stood out about the group.

Discussion Focus: Tell members that this and all subsequent groups will end by asking each member to comment on one thing that stood out for them in the group. Because the group leaders are part of the group, they also summarize, but they go last. Comments by the leaders are intended to reinforce behaviors they observed in the group or how certain issues were discussed and dealt with by the group members Start the next two wrap-ups by calling on someone who volunteers. If no one comments, ask one member to start.

What Was Group Like?: *"Now that we have completed the first group session, what we would like to do is go around asking everyone how it felt to be in the group today, particularly in relation to what you expected."*

What Stood Out?: Have each group member and the leaders comment on one thing that stood out in the group. *"We have talked about a lot of things in group today. What one thing stood out?"*

Remind Group Members: (1) to attend all group sessions, (2) to call if they cannot make a session, (3) to continue to use the self-monitoring logs and bring them and the homework exercise to the next session, and (4) that one of the leaders will call the day before group to remind everyone about the next group.

POSTGROUP DISCUSSION

- The postgroup discussion typically takes about 5–10 minutes.
- Discuss what happened in the group, both good and less good things.
- Group leaders should make notes about what they want to highlight in the next session and about anything notable about group members.
- Prior to the next group session, for each group member prepare a Client Handout 4.7: BSCQ Profile of high-risk situations for alcohol or drug use.

Objectives, Procedures, Client Handouts, Pregroup Planning, and Sample Round-Robin Discussions
Group Session 2

SESSION OBJECTIVES

- Review members' progress.
- Identify high-risk situations for members based on homework and BSCQ.
- Give homework and instructions for Session 3.

SESSION PROCEDURES

- Introduce session.
- Review and discuss members' completed self-monitoring logs; copy or record data.
- Review and discuss members' answers to Identifying Triggers homework exercise.
- Give members BSCQ feedback profiles and discuss relationship to Identifying Triggers homework answers.
- Have members complete Where Are You Now Scale (Client Handout 3.6) and compare their answers with their answers at the assessment.
- End session: Ask what stood out about session; remind members to do their homework.

CLIENT HANDOUTS

- Exercise: Developing Options and Action Plans (Client Handout 4.8)
- Have the group members' Where Are You Now Scale for them to check where they are at this session.

PREGROUP PLANNING

- Group leaders review what happened at the last group.
- Group leaders decide who will take the lead on which discussion topics (e.g., self-monitoring, homework).
- Prepare and have BSCQ personalized feedback profiles for members based on assessment interview.
- Have new homework for members (Client Handout 4.8).
- Have group members complete Where Are You Now Scale.

(cont.)

ROUND-ROBIN DISCUSSION

Topic: Review Members' Completed Self-Monitoring Logs for Their Alcohol or Drug Use since Session 1 (Alcohol: Client Handout 3.2; Drug: Client Handout 3.3)

Discussion Focus

- The discussion can start with a group leader saying, *"Let's go over the self-monitoring logs and look at everybody's alcohol and drug use in the past week."* Follow up by asking a member to begin the discussion, *"[**Insert client name**], give us a general picture of what your alcohol or drug use was like this past week."*
- **Note to Group Leaders:** Unless relevant, avoid specific details of a client's drinking or drug use (i.e., do not have members present a day-by-day description, as this takes too much time and usually is not that informative).
- If major changes have occurred or if a member handled a difficult situation and did not use, the group leaders can ask the group how they feel about the group member's change.

ROUND-ROBIN DISCUSSION

Topic: Identification of High-Risk Trigger Situations for Alcohol or Drug Use (Reading: Client Handout 4.5; Exercise: Client Handout 4.6)

Discussion Focus

- Discuss the reading and exercise on identification of high-risk trigger situations for alcohol and drug use, including taking a realistic perspective on change (i.e., Mt. Change) and viewing slips as learning experiences.
- Probe group members' understanding of the reading on identifying triggers of alcohol and drug use (Client Handout 4.5). There are two parts to this exercise: (1) identifying and evaluating personal high-risk triggers to alcohol or drug use and (2) a relapse prevention approach to change and taking a realistic perspective on change.
- A good question leaders can ask about the reading is, *"The reading talks about taking a long-term view of change and that there might be some bumps in the road. What do you think is meant by this?"*
- Another topic for members is to have them discuss the *Mt. Change* diagram (see picture in Client Handout 4.5). For example, the leaders could say, *"What would you say is the major message of Mt. Change in terms of dealing with your alcohol or drug use?"*
- Have clients select and discuss one of their two identified triggers from the exercise: *"Let's go around and have each member tell us about one of the high-risk trigger situations they described for their alcohol or drug use."*
- **Note to Group Leaders:** As part of this discussion, look for and acknowledge commonalities among members in terms of high-risk situations. Leaders can recognize commonalities with reflections: *"So it looks like a high-risk situation for both Bill and Mary is when they are angry. Who else feels at risk when they experience strong emotions?"*

Note to Group Leaders: With regard to the reading, members should recognize that for many people change might be associated with slips but that the important thing if a slip occurs is to continue up the mountain. However, it is also essential that the leaders not convey a self-fulfilling prophecy to the group (i.e., that they will have slips). A good way of presenting the concept is to have one of the group leaders ask, *"Why do schools have fire drills?"* Most members come up with the obvious response,

(cont.)

"So you're better prepared if a fire occurs." The leaders can follow this with, *"That's the same idea here. Hopefully you won't have any slips, but it makes sense to be prepared in case they occur."*

It is also important for group members to recognize that, if slips occur, they should interrupt them early and learn from them. If a group member brings up a slip in group, one of the leaders can say:

- *"Mary, can you tell the group what you think triggered the slip that occurred last Wednesday. What was different about Wednesday?"*
- *"How have others in the group handled a slip?"*
- *"What is another way of looking at a slip than as a failure?"*

ROUND-ROBIN DISCUSSION

Topic: Review Brief Situational Confidence Questionnaire (BSCQ) Feedback and Relationship to High-Risk Triggers (Client Handout 4.7)

Discussion Focus

- Give members copies of their BSCQ Profiles (Client Handout 4.7) that were prepared based on the BSCQ they completed at the assessment.
- Have group members compare their BSCQ profiles with their two individual high-risk situations from the Identifying Triggers exercise. Ask how the two high-risk triggers in their homework exercise relate to their generic BSCQ profile.
- For a majority of members, their BSCQ profiles and triggers from the Identifying Triggers exercise will be similar.
- Point out for those whose BSCQ profiles and triggers are similar that the general BSCQ profile names are a shorthand that can help them more easily identify situations that could trigger future alcohol or drug use and that they should be vigilant in such situations. One of the leaders can ask, *"Why is it important to know the types of situations in which you might be at risk of heavy drinking or drug use?"*

Note to Group Leaders: In the discussion it will help members to recall their high-risk situations if the leaders label the members' BSCQ profiles with shorthand names of the different BSCQ profiles listed in Table 4.2 (e.g., Good Time profile; Negative Affective profile; Testing Personal Control profile).

ROUND-ROBIN DISCUSSION

Topic: Review of Members' Completed Where Are You Now Scales (Client Handout 3.6)

Discussion Focus

- Give members the Where Are You Now Scale completed at the assessment and ask them to answer the same questions again but for Session 2.
- *"When you first came in, we asked each of you to rate how serious you thought your alcohol or drug use was on a 10-point scale. How would each of you rate your alcohol or drug use today on that same scale, where 1 = the most serious concern and 10 = no longer a concern?"*
- Have members try to remember what number characterized where they were at the assessment interview on this scale.
- Ask members, *"How did you go from a [**# at Assessment**] to a [**# now**]?"*

(cont.)

- This scaling question is a motivational interviewing technique that allows members to give voice to changes they have made.
  - ♦ As part of this discussion, look for and acknowledge commonalities among members, and encourage them to be supportive of changes others are making.
  - ♦ For members who have not changed, the leaders can ask, *"What would you need to do to move up a number or two?"* or *"What kinds of things have gotten in the way of your changing?"*

DEVELOPING NEW OPTIONS AND ACTION PLANS HOMEWORK ASSIGNMENT FOR SESSION 3 (CLIENT HANDOUT 4.8)

Discussion Focus

- Give each member Client Handout 4.8, which asks them to develop new options and action plans for the two high-risk trigger situations they described in the exercise on identifying high-risk triggers associated with their alcohol or drug use.
- Group leaders can say to members, *"This exercise is intended to help you learn how to handle those situations you identified as high-risk triggers by doing things other than using alcohol or drugs. This exercise will ask you not only to come up with some new options you could implement but also to evaluate how well they might work to help you resist using alcohol or drugs. Then you decide which are your best options and develop plans for how to put them into action. The exercise should take about 10 minutes to complete."*
- Finally, ask group members to complete the exercise at home and bring it to Session 3. Tell them that next week each member will be asked to talk about the options and action plans he or she developed for one of their two high-risk trigger situations.

ROUND-ROBIN DISCUSSION

Topic: End of Session, Wrap-Up, and What Stood Out

Discussion Focus

- **What Stood Out?:** Have each group member and the leaders comment on one thing that stood out in the group: *"We have talked about a lot of things in group today. What one thing stood out?"*
- **Remind Group Members:** (1) to attend all group sessions, (2) to call if they cannot make a session, (3) to continue to use the self-monitoring logs and bring them and the homework exercise to the next session, and (4) that one of the leaders will call the day before group to remind everyone about the next group.

Postgroup Discussion

- The postgroup discussion typically takes about 5–10 minutes.
- Discuss what happened in the group, both the good things and less good things.
- Group leaders should make notes about what they want to highlight in the next session and about anything notable about the behavior of group members.

Objectives, Procedures, Client Handouts, Pregroup Planning, and Sample Round-Robin Discussions
Group Session 3

SESSION OBJECTIVES

- Review members' progress.
- Discuss members' change plans.
- Discuss new options and action plans for the high-risk trigger situations.
- Give homework and instructions for Session 4.

SESSION PROCEDURES

- Introduce session.
- Review and discuss members' completed self-monitoring logs; copy or record data.
- Have members complete second BSCQ.
- Review and discuss members' answers to homework exercise "Developing New Options and Action Plans."
- Discuss possible opportunities for testing options before Session 4.
- End session: Ask what stood out about session; remind members to do their homework.

CLIENT HANDOUTS

- Homework: Request for Additional Sessions form (Client Handout 4.10)
- Homework: Goal Evaluation form (Client Handout 3.4 for members with an abstinence goal; Client Handout 3.5 for members with a low-risk limited drinking goal)
- BSCQ form (Appendix D) to be completed in session by each group member

PREGROUP PLANNING

- Group leaders review what happened at the last group.
- Group leaders decide who will take the lead on which discussion topics (e.g., self-monitoring, homework).
- Have new homework for members.
  - ◆ Request for Additional Sessions form (Client Handout 4.10)
  - ◆ Goal Evaluation form (Client Handout 3.4 for members with an abstinence goal; Client Handout 3.5 for members with a low-risk limited drinking goal)
- Have a new BSCQ form for each group member to complete in this group session (Appendix D).

(cont.)

ROUND-ROBIN DISCUSSION

*Topic: Review Members' Completed Self-Monitoring Logs for Their Alcohol or Drug Use since Session
2 (Alcohol: Client Handout 3.2; Drug: Client Handout 3.3)*

Discussion Focus

- The discussion can start with a group leader saying, *"Let's go over the self-monitoring logs and look
  at everybody's alcohol and drug use in the past week."* Follow up by asking a member to begin the
  discussion: *"***[Insert client name]**, *give us a general picture of what your alcohol or drug use was like
  this past week."*
- **Note to Group Leaders:** Unless relevant, avoid specific details of a client's drinking or drug use (i.e.,
  do not have members present a day-by-day description, as this takes too much time and usually is
  not that informative).
- If major changes have occurred or if a member handled a difficult situation and did not use, the
  group leaders can ask the group how they feel about the group member's change.

ROUND-ROBIN DISCUSSION

*Topic: Discuss New Homework Exercise on Developing Options and Action Plans (Client Handout
4.8)*

Discussion Focus

- Ask each member to discuss the options and action plan for one of his or her two identified trigger
  situations from the homework.
- The goal is to use a motivational interviewing approach to have group members give voice to their
  change plans.
- *"What kinds of options and action plans did you develop for your high-risk situations?"*
- *"Which option did you select as the most realistic to implement and why?"*
- **Note to Group Leaders:** Tell members that it is important, when possible, to break action plans into
  small steps so that progress can be identified.

  Ask each member, *"What trigger situations can you anticipate occurring between now and the next
  session in which you could put into practice your options and action plans?"* [This question is used
  to identify possible future high-risk situations that group members might encounter and ways to deal
  with those situations in advance.]

IN-SESSION ASSIGNMENT

Complete Brief Situational Confidence Questionnaire (Appendix D)

Discussion Focus

- Give each member a BSCQ to complete during the session and tell him or her, *"This form assesses
  how confident you are at the present time that you can resist the urge to drink heavily or use drugs.
  At the assessment you completed this form, and we want you to complete it again. Next week we
  will discuss and compare your answers today with your answers when you first came in."*

(cont.)

GOAL EVALUATION FORM HOMEWORK ASSIGNMENT FOR SESSION 4 (ABSTINENCE: CLIENT HANDOUT 3.4; GOAL CHOICE: CLIENT HANDOUT 3.5)

Discussion Focus

- Give each member either Client Handout 3.4 (members with an abstinence goal) or Client Handout 3.5 (members with a low-risk limited drinking goal) and ask them to complete the form at home and bring it to the next session.

  "This is the same form you completed and brought into Session 1. We would like you to fill it out again and bring it to the next session, where we will compare your answers with your answers when you first came in."

REQUEST FOR ADDITIONAL SESSIONS FORM HOMEWORK ASSIGNMENT FOR SESSION 4 (CLIENT HANDOUT 4.10)

Discussion Focus

- Give members the Request for Additional Sessions form (Client Handout 4.10) and ask them to complete the form at home and bring it to the next session.
- *"As was mentioned at the assessment, next week will be our last group session. Some people will feel they do not need any additional sessions as they have made sufficient progress, whereas others will want to continue in treatment. Additional sessions will occur as individual sessions rather than in groups. On this form you can indicate whether you want additional sessions, and if so, how many and what you would like to accomplish. If you want more sessions, we can discuss your request individually after the group next week."*

ROUND-ROBIN DISCUSSION

End of Session, Wrap-Up, and What Stood Out

Have each group member and the leaders comment on one thing that stood out in the group. *"We have talked about a lot of things in group today. What one thing stood out?"*

Remind Group Members: (1) to attend all group sessions, (2) to call if they cannot make a session, (3) to continue to use the self-monitoring logs and bring them and the homework exercises to the next session, and (4) that one of the leaders will call the day before group to remind everyone about the next group.

POSTGROUP DISCUSSION

- The postgroup discussion typically takes about 5–10 minutes.
- Discuss what happened in the group, both the good things and less good things.
- Group leaders should make notes about what they want to highlight in the next session and anything notable about the behavior of group members.
- For all members, prepare personalized comparative BSCQ profiles (assessment and Session 3) of high-risk situations for alcohol or drug use (Client Handout 4.9).
- For all members, prepare a personalized comparative (assessment to Session 3) feedback form of their alcohol or drug use (Alcohol: Client Handout 4.3; Drug: Client Handout 4.4).

Objectives, Procedures, Client Handouts, Pregroup Planning, and Sample Round-Robin Discussions
Group Session 4

SESSION OBJECTIVES

- Review members' progress.
- Revisit and review members' motivation and goals.
- Discuss end of treatment and aftercare call, or schedule further sessions.

SESSION PROCEDURES

- Introduce session.
- Review and discuss members' completed self-monitoring logs in relation to goal; copy or record data.
- Discuss opportunities for testing options since last session and the outcomes.
- Give members their personalized feedback comparisons of alcohol use (Client Handout 4.3) or drug use (Client Handout 4.4) over the course of treatment and discuss.
- Revisit goals, revise if necessary.
- Revisit decisional balance exercise, revise if necessary.
- Give members the BSCQ comparison (Client Handout 4.9) of assessment and Session 3 answers and discuss.
- Revisit and review members' understanding of the Mt. Change diagram and taking a realistic long-term perspective on change.
- Have members complete the Where Are You Now Scale and compare it with their assessment and Session 2 answers.
- Discuss Request for Additional Sessions form (Client Handout 4.10) completed as homework by members.
- Ensure that the members know how to contact the program if they need further treatment. Also, mention that one of the group leaders will contact them in about 1 month to check on how they are doing and whether anything else is needed.
- End session: Ask what stood out about the session.

PREGROUP PLANNING

- Group leaders review what happened at the last group.
- Group leaders decide what discussion topics (e.g., self-monitoring, homework) each will take the lead on for this session.
- Have a copy for each member of his or her BSCQ comparative feedback profiles (assessment and Session 3; Client Handout 4.9).
- Have a copy for each member of their comparative (assessment to Session 3) feedback profiles for alcohol use (Client Handout 4.3) or drug use (Client Handout 4.4).
- Have the Where Are You Now Scale for members to complete again.

(cont.)

ROUND-ROBIN DISCUSSION

*Review Members' Completed Self-Monitoring Logs for Their Alcohol or Drug Use since Session 3
(Alcohol: Client Handout 3.2; Drug: Client Handout 3.3)*

Discussion Focus

- The discussion can start with a group leader saying, *"Let's go over the self-monitoring logs and look at everybody's alcohol and drug use in the past week."* Follow up by asking a member to begin the discussion: *"[**Insert client name**], give us a general picture of what your alcohol or drug use was like this past week."*
- **Note to Group Leaders:** Unless relevant, avoid specific details of a client's drinking or drug use (i.e., do not have members present a day-by-day description, as this takes too much time and usually is not that informative).
- If major changes have occurred or if a member handled a difficult situation and did not use, the group leaders can ask the group how they feel about the group member's change.

ROUND-ROBIN DISCUSSION

Topic: Discussion of Comparative Personalized Feedback about Changes in Alcohol or Drug Use Before and During Treatment (Alcohol Use: Client Handout 4.3; Drug Use: Client Handout 4.4)

Discussion Focus: Alcohol Use

- Give members copies of their alcohol feedback handouts (Client Handout 4.3). This feedback form allows members to give voice to changes in their alcohol use.
- *"These handouts display your alcohol use when you first came in and over the course of treatment. The first graph compares how frequently each one of you drank during the 90 days preceding your treatment and how frequently you drank during the time you were in the program up to last week. The second graph compares how much you drank per day during the 90 days preceding your treatment and during the time you were in the program up through last week. In looking at these two graphs, how would each of you say your drinking has changed?"*

Discussion Focus: Drug Use

- Give members copies of their drug feedback handouts (Client Handout 4.4). This feedback form allows members give voice to changes in their drug use.
- *"These handouts display your drug use when you first came in and over the course of treatment. The graph compares how frequently each one of you used drugs during the 90 days preceding your treatment and during the time you were in the program up through last week. In looking at these graphs, how would each of you say your drug use has changed?"*

(cont.)

ROUND-ROBIN DISCUSSION

Topic: Comparative (Assessment and Session 3) Goal Evaluations (Abstinence: Client Handout 3.4; Goal Choice: Client Handout 3.5)

Discussion Focus

- This evaluation form was handed out as homework at the last session. The discussion will focus on members' alcohol or drug use during treatment and how it relates to their goals and possible changes in their goals.
- *"First, let's look at your new goal and compare it with your goal when you first came in. What changes, if any, have you made and what led to these changes?"*
- *"Looking at your self-monitoring logs, how consistent is your recent alcohol and drug use with your second goal statement?"* For members whose behavior is not consistent with their goals, ask the group, *"Who has some ideas about why things haven't been working for* [**insert member's name**]*?"*
- *"How and why have your importance and confidence ratings changed?"*
- If change has occurred, ask, *"How does the change feel and how has it affected your confidence level compared with when you first came in to treatment?"*
- The leaders can get other members to comment by asking, *"Who else has had similar experiences?"*
- Supportive comments from other members about members who have changed can be elicited by asking, *"Both Bill and Mary have made some major changes. How do others feel about what they've done?"*
- Finally, group leaders can ask, *"What do members have to do to maintain the changes they have made?"*

ROUND-ROBIN DISCUSSION

Topic: Revisiting the Decisional Balance Exercise

Discussion Focus

- Have members look back at their decisional balance exercises from Session 1 and revisit what they wrote down. The discussion relates to any additions or changes in members' answers from Session 1.
- *"Let's look at the decisional balance exercise each of you completed at the start of treatment. Are there any new good or less good things that you did not identify earlier?"*
- *"Have any of the original good or less good things proved to be different from what you expected, and why?"* [Often members will report that anticipated negative consequences of changing did not occur after all.]

ROUND-ROBIN DISCUSSION

Topic: Discuss Changes in the Brief Situational Confidence Questionnaire (BSCQ; Client Handout 4.9)

Discussion Focus

- Review the BSCQ personalized profiles of members' high-risk situations for alcohol or drug use completed at assessment and at Session 3.

(cont.)

- Give members feedback comparing their first and second BSCQ profiles. Using a motivational counseling style allows group members to give voice to changes they have experienced in their confidence to resist the urge to drink heavily or use drugs.
- *"What changes have you noticed in the situations you previously identified as high risk?"*
- *"What led to your change in confidence?"*

ROUND-ROBIN DISCUSSION

Topic: Discussion of the Implementation of Options to Deal With the High-Risk Trigger Situations since the Last Session

Discussion Focus

- *"Who can tell us about an opportunity they had to put one of their action plans to work and how it turned out?"*

ROUND-ROBIN DISCUSSION

Topic: Revisit Mt. Change and Relapse Prevention

Discussion Focus

Revisit the concept of taking a realistic, long-term perspective on change. Look for statements that change may be slow and that if a slip occurs one can learn from it, get up, and keep on going.

- *"Think back to Session 2 when we talked about Mt. Change and taking a long-term perspective on change. Based on our previous discussions and group meetings, what does taking a realistic perspective on change mean to you now?"*
- *"How are you going to accomplish this?"*

ROUND-ROBIN DISCUSSION

Topic: Review Members' Where Are You Now Scale Answers over Treatment (Client Handout 3.6)

Discussion Focus

- Give members the Where Are You Now Scale completed at the assessment and Session 2 and ask them to answer the same questions again for Session 4.
- *"When you first came in, and again at the second session, we asked each of you to rate how serious you thought your alcohol or drug use was on a 10-point scale. How would each of you rate your alcohol or drug use today on that same scale, where 1 = the most serious concern and 10 = no longer a concern?"*
- Have members try to remember what number characterized where they were at the assessment interview on this scale and what number they put down at Session 2. Then ask, *"How did each of you get from where you were when you first entered treatment to where you are now, and how do you feel about this?"*
- Look for and acknowledge commonalities, and encourage members to praise others for change.

(cont.)

REQUEST FOR ADDITIONAL SESSIONS

"Before we wrap up, last week we gave you a Request for Additional Sessions form to fill out and bring in today. For those of you who are requesting additional sessions, we'll meet with you individually after the group to discuss it."

ROUND-ROBIN DISCUSSION

End of Session, Wrap-Up, and What Stood Out

Have each group member and the leaders comment on one thing that stood out in the group. *"We have talked about a lot of things in group today. What one thing stood out?"*
Remind Group Members: *"One of us will be calling each of you in about a month to ask about your progress and to schedule additional sessions if needed."*

POSTGROUP DISCUSSION

- The postgroup discussion typically takes about 5–10 minutes.
- Discuss what happened in the group as a whole, both good things and less good things, and what lessons the leaders can take away from the entire group experience.

Introduction to Groups

RESEARCH SHOWS THAT GROUPS ARE AS EFFECTIVE AS INDIVIDUAL THERAPY.

GROUPS GIVE YOU AN OPPORTUNITY TO

- Share your experiences with others.
- Learn how others deal with their problems.
- Receive support from those who have similar problems.
- Help others deal with their problems.

HOW TO BENEFIT FROM GROUPS

ATTEND ALL SESSIONS: Attend all sessions and arrive on time. If for some reason you cannot make the group, call in advance and tell the group leaders.

DO THE READINGS AND HOMEWORK ASSIGNMENTS: You will be given readings, homework exercises, and self-monitoring logs to complete at home and bring back to the groups. This helps use the time in groups more efficiently. The assignments and self-monitoring logs will be discussed in the group.

PARTICIPATE: To get the most out of the groups, members need to participate during every group session and take turns speaking.

SELF-DISCLOSE: Use the group to help you with your own problems by sharing with the rest of the group.

WORK TOGETHER: The group accomplishes more when members work together, much like a sports team.

GROUP RULES

CONFIDENTIALITY: What is discussed in the group is not repeated outside the group.

DO NOT SOCIALIZE OUTSIDE OF THE GROUP

AVOID DISRUPTIVE BEHAVIORS

NO ALCOHOL OR DRUG USE: It is important not to use alcohol or drugs before coming to the group.

TURN CELL PHONES OFF DURING GROUPS

PART III

Conducting and Managing Groups

Pregroup Planning, Group Cohesion, and Difficult Situations and Clients

CHAPTER 6

Building Group Cohesion
Music Comes from the Group

There is highly persuasive evidence that pregroup
preparation expedites the course of group psychotherapy.
—YALOM AND LESZCZ (2005, p. 294)

In group psychotherapy, the relationship between the leader
and the group member seems to be less important than the
group members' relationships with each other as a group.
—SCHOENHOLTZ-READ (1994, p. 157)

GROUP PREPARATION AND PLANNING

Pregroup planning and preparation are critical to the retention of members in groups and contribute to members' satisfaction, group cohesion, and group outcomes (Burlingame, Fuhriman, & Johnson, 2001; MacKenzie, 1994; Rosenberg & Zimet, 1995; Satterfield, 1994; Yalom & Leszcz, 2005). Research has shown that pregroup planning has many benefits, including reducing dropout rates, increasing attendance, increasing self-disclosure by group members, increasing group cohesion, facilitating early group participation, reducing overall apprehension about groups, and, most important, increasing motivation to change (reviewed in Piper, 1993; Rosenberg & Zimet, 1995; Satterfield, 1994; Yalom & Leszcz, 2005).

Selling the Group

As discussed in Chapter 1, although research has shown that groups generally are as effective as their individual-therapy counterparts, many clients nevertheless believe that groups are not as effective as individual therapy (Yalom & Leszcz, 2005). Because several studies (Budman et al., 1988; Hofmann & Suvak, 2006), including the one in this book (L. C. Sobell et al., 2009), have reported that clients overwhelmingly prefer individual to group therapy, it is important to market groups to clients.

When possible, group leaders should meet with potential members prior to the first group session to explain how groups work and to address concerns about participating in groups. Discussions with potential group members typically include (1) how the group works; (2) the role and expectations of group members (e.g., to learn from their peers, to be supportive of other members, to provide constructive feedback); (3) group rules; and (4) the importance of all members participating at each group. Because most clients can be expected to be ambivalent about attending group therapy, providing information about the benefits of groups and expectations of members should be done in a manner that is consistent with motivational interviewing principles (Miller & Rollnick, 2002). Potential members can be given a handout about the benefits of groups (see Client Handout 5.1 for a sample), including practical information about the logistics of groups such as parking or who to contact if a problem arises).

Group rules are intended to shape appropriate group behaviors, promote positive group norms, and reduce clients' anxieties. The group rules most commonly advocated and their rationales were listed in Table 5.3 (Bieling et al., 2006; MacKenzie, 1994; Yalom & Leszcz, 2005). Among the most important are attending group on time, maintaining confidentiality, not using alcohol or illicit drugs before group, not talking about group members who are not present, participating regularly, not socializing outside of groups, completing homework assignments and bringing them to group, and exhibiting appropriate behaviors in groups (i.e., no yelling, no profanity, no use of cell phone during groups, no talking over one another).

Preparation Prior to Each Session

Pregroup planning includes everything from making sure the room where the group will meet is ready and has the right number of chairs (MacKenzie, 1994) to discussing issues regarding specific members. Generally, pregroup preparation and planning should take about 15 to 20 minutes. To facilitate nonverbal communication in the group, it has been recommended that cotherapists sit opposite one another (Yalom & Leszcz, 2005). Before the group starts, when the chairs are being arranged, the group leaders can place their handouts or a clipboard on the chairs where they will be sitting. As described in Table 6.1, prior to each group the cotherapists should complete several tasks (e.g., discussing the group's objectives; determining how responsibilities will be shared, such as who will keep track of time spent on different tasks; discussing members' progress and special issues, such as how to better engage silent members; housekeeping tasks, such as having sign-in sheets and relevant homework assignments). Finally, when the group is ready to begin, empty chairs should be removed from the circle.

TABLE 6.1. Tasks for Cotherapists Prior to Each Group Therapy Session

- Specify the objectives and tasks to be accomplished and the topics to be discussed during the session.
- Decide who is going to start and end the group and who will take responsibility for starting the discussions related to specific session topics and homework exercises. For open groups, it is a good idea to think about general discussion topics in advance so there is some structure.
- Review notes from the previous session to identify topics that were to be followed up and discussed at the next group session. Also, briefly review each group member's participation in and progress over the course of group sessions. If therapists use an ongoing logbook to make their postgroup notes, it will be easier to recall what happened in the previous session.
- Make sure that relevant paperwork needed for the session is available (e.g., sign-in sheets, confidentiality forms, group rules, handouts).
- Arrange chairs in a circle and have only enough for the number of anticipated participants plus the group leaders.

Postgroup Discussions

Postgroup discussions are also important (Dies, 1994; Yalom & Leszcz, 2005) and usually last 10 to 15 minutes. Topics that can be discussed include how the group went and any concerns or problems that arose from the group discussions. If something did not go as planned (e.g., discussion of planned exercise), the cotherapists can discuss why and how to handle it next time. Based on the postgroup discussion, a plan for the next session can be developed, including identifying members and topics to address (Heimberg & Becker, 2002). If trainees are present, the postgroup discussion provides an opportunity for them to ask questions. Last, issues that need to be followed up or addressed in the next session should be written in an ongoing group log so they can be recalled prior to the next group meeting.

GROUP: A LIVING, LEARNING HALL OF MIRRORS

The group experience is a key part of the learning process for group members. Discussing one's successes or difficulties in groups allows other members to learn from such interactions, to be supportive, and to offer suggestions for change. In this sense groups can be thought of as a *living, learning hall of mirrors* in which members have the opportunity to practice behaviors, see how they are perceived by others, and get feedback, both positive and negative, from other group members (R. R. Dies, personal communication, February 19, 1996; Dies, 1992, 1994; MacKenzie, 1994). Groups provide a context in which real-life experiences and situations can be simulated in safe circumstances with feedback from others (e.g., *"Bill, could you tell the group how the meeting went last week that you and your wife had with your children's counselor?"*). Group members, in contrast to the group leaders, can provide different perspectives on members' behaviors and offer social support and peer pressure to encourage members to change. Groups also provide an opportunity to learn from other members through observational or vicarious learning. In discussing the benefits of groups, Satterfield said, "Group interactions also provide a natural arena to test social hypotheses, practice newly acquired skills, and create a 'therapeutic' mirror' showing the objective social consequences of a patient's actions and beliefs" (1994, p. 186).

MUSIC COMES FROM THE GROUP: THERAPISTS AS ORCHESTRA CONDUCTORS

As discussed in the Acknowledgments section, several years ago we attended two workshops presented by Dr. Robert Dies. During the trainings, he discussed two important concepts that we feel are key to understanding how to successfully manage groups. The first, *Think Group*, is intended to help therapists remember that the group itself is an agent of change and not to do individual therapy in group settings (also see p. 86 in Dies, 1994). The second concept—*Music Comes from the Group* and *Therapists as Conductors*—relates to the role of therapists in developing interactions among group members. In group therapy, the leaders' task is to get the music to come from the group, which involves the members accepting responsibility for change and group processes driving the change. As we discuss subsequently, the concepts of *Music Comes from the Group* and *Therapists as Conductors* are straightforward and visually communicative. Over the years, we have found these two simple and eloquent concepts to be very effective in communicating to trainees how to manage and think about group processes.

Most group therapy experts recommend having two leaders, or cotherapists. Cotherapists can be likened to orchestra conductors, with group members being the instruments composing the orchestra. The leaders' task is to get group members to work together, helping each other change. To apply the analogy *Music Comes from the Group*, an orchestra sounds good only when the instruments play together appropriately. In group therapy, for the music to success-fully come from the group, the members should be doing most of the talking (i.e., playing the music) and interacting to facilitate change. Sometimes the conductor (i.e., group leader) will want to hear from the entire orchestra and will invite the whole group to respond (e.g., *"Who else can identify with what Bill has said?"*). At other times, the conductor/group leader will want a particular section of the orchestra (e.g., trombones) to play (e.g., *"Bill, can you help Mary out?"*) or will want to hear a different instrument (e.g., *"Bill, we haven't heard from you today. Can you offer Mary some suggestions for how she can handle her situation at work?"*). At other times, the conductor/group leader may hear one instrument/group member play badly and will ask another instrument/group member to demonstrate how to play the part (e.g., *"Bill, that is one way of handling things. Who can offer Mary another suggestion?"*). Last, on rare occasions, a conductor/group leader might feel that the sound from the entire orchestra is not good. When this happens, the conductor/group leader may put down the baton and call a time-out, saying, *"A lot is happening in group right now, and I'm not comfortable with what I'm hearing. Let's stop and talk about what's going on."* The ultimate goal of the orchestra conductor/group leader is to enable the members of the orchestra/group to work together (i.e., cohesion) to produce a harmonious sound.

COHESION: A POTENT FORCE IN GROUP THERAPY

Cohesion, a dynamic process that fluctuates over time, has been associated with positive out-comes (Beal, Cohen, Burke, & McLendon, 2003; Burlingame et al., 2001; Rose, 1990; Satter-field, 1994; Tschuschke, Hess, & MacKenzie, 2002) and with several key group attributes (Bur-lingame et al., 2001; Satterfield, 1994; Stokes, 1983; Yalom & Leszcz, 2005). Those attributes include: (1) productivity, (2) participation in and out of the group, (3) self-disclosure, (4) risk taking, (5) regular attendance, (6) pregroup preparation, (7) feedback, and (8) compliance with homework exercises. According to Yalom and Leszcz (2005), "group cohesiveness is not only a potent therapeutic force in its own right. It is a precondition for other therapeutic factors to function optimally" (p. 55). For these reasons, cohesion can be viewed as the *glue that holds the group together* and as a sine qua non for effective group therapy.

Building Cohesion in Groups

To develop group cohesion, group leaders need to look for and highlight similarities among members based on information from the assessments (e.g., types of problems clients have) and from interactions during group sessions (e.g., how clients have handled or avoided problems). Group leaders can use commonalities among members (1) to draw more group members into the discussion, (2) to demonstrate that others have had similar experiences, and (3) to prompt members to share how they have handled similar problems. Good group preparation by the leaders is important for developing group cohesion. For example, if two or more members have undergone a recent divorce and the topic comes up in group, one of the group leaders can say, *"If I recall, Mary is not the only one who has gone through a divorce. Who can share with Mary how they've dealt with this?"* A leader could also ask, *"Who else has had similar experiences?"* or *"Who else can identify with what Mary is feeling?"* Although some group members will mention similarities and differences with other clients, at times the group leaders will have to prompt the group (*"Who can offer Mary some advice about how they've dealt with being served with divorce papers and having to look for an attorney?"*). Although clients tell different stories, there are common themes therapists can identify and ask others to comment on (*"Perhaps others who have dealt with* [insert type of problem] *can share with Mary how they handled the situation?"*).

Building group cohesion starts at the first group session, in which clients begin by talking about relatively safe topics (e.g., introducing themselves, describing their expectations from the group). As clients reveal their thoughts and feelings, it is important for the therapists to establish a favorable climate by commenting on the similarities and reinforcing clients for relating to each other and sharing their experiences. For example, following a member's appropriate participation, the leader can say, *"Mary, that is exactly what we are looking for. We want each of you to share your experiences with the group."* It is also important that the leaders ensure that all members have an opportunity to participate. As illustrated in Chapter 5, round-robin discussions can be used to ensure that all group members participate regularly.

Cohesion: The Glue That Holds Groups Together

Burlingame and colleagues (2001, p. 373) have defined cohesion as "the therapeutic relationship in group psychotherapy emerging from the aggregate of member–leader, member–member, and member–group relationships." Yalom and Leszcz (2005) consider group cohesion to be one of the most important therapeutic factors in group therapy. In his book *Group Dynamics*, Forsyth (2006) asserts that "a cohesive group is a unified one, so members literally 'stick together'" (p. 136).

In sports psychology, group cohesion is also very important. Sports psychologists talk about cohesion as integrating the members of a team (Moran, 2004). Interestingly, the concept has been used to explain the success of sports teams that were not expected to do well. Two key examples are the "Miracle on Ice" U.S. men's hockey team that won the 1980 Olympic gold medal and the 1997 Florida Marlins baseball team, a group of very young and inexperienced players who started performing well, believed in themselves and in each other, and went on to win the World Series.

The Group Is Greater Than the Sum of Its Parts

The importance of group processes is summed up in the observation that more can be accomplished by members working together as a group than as individuals (Forsyth, 2006; MacKenzie, 1994). Burlingame and colleagues (2001) have summarized and discussed six empirically supported principles related to therapeutic relationships in groups. These six principles are reproduced from the original article in Table 6.2. What is striking is that many of the *member-to-member* and *leader-to-member* interactions discussed by Burlingame and colleagues are con-

TABLE 6.2. Empirically Supported Principles Regarding the Therapeutic Relationship in Group Treatment

Principle 1: Pregroup preparation sets treatment expectations, defines group rules, and instructs members in appropriate roles and skills needed for effective group participation and group cohesion.

Principle 2: The group leaders should establish clarity regarding group processes in early sessions since higher levels of structure are thought to lead to higher levels of group disclosure and cohesion.

Principle 3: Group leaders who model real-time observations, effectively guide interpersonal feedback, and maintain a moderate level of control and affiliation may positively impact group cohesion.

Principle 4: The timing and delivery of feedback should be pivotal considerations for group leaders as they facilitate this relationship-building process.

Principle 5: The group leaders' presence not only affects the relationship with individual members, but also with all group members as they vicariously experience the leaders' manner of relating, and thus learn the importance of managing one's own emotional presence in the service of others.

Principle 6: A primary objective of the group leaders should be to facilitate group members' emotional expression, the responsiveness of others to that expression, and the shared meaning derived from that expression.

Note. From Burlingame, Fuhriman, and Johnson (2001, p. 375). Copyright 2001 by the Division of Psychotherapy (29), American Psychological Association. Reprinted by permission.

sistent with the cognitive-behavioral strategies and the motivational interviewing approach used in the GSC treatment model. In retrospect, the many parallels between the GSC approach and group processes might explain why we were able to successfully integrate cognitive-behavioral techniques and a motivational interviewing counseling approach into a group therapy format. In the next two paragraphs, words and phrases common to the Burlingame and colleagues study and the GSC treatment model are italicized.

Member-to-Member Interactions

Several member-to-member interactions have been shown to increase group cohesion and contribute to successful groups (Burlingame et al., 2001): (1) being *supportive* of each other's changing; (2) responding *empathically* (i.e., with genuine regard); (3) giving *feedback* to others *in a nonjudgmental manner* (minimizing negativity is more likely to get members to accept feedback and to be *less resistant to change*); (4) members *assuming responsibility for their own change*; and (5) *complying with structured behavioral activities* in groups (e.g., homework exercises and self-monitoring logs foster commonalities in terms of disclosures and shared feedback about ways to handle problems, all of which lead to greater group cohesion).

Leader-to-Member Interactions

With respect to leader-to-member interactions, the following have been shown to produce positive results in groups (Burlingame et al., 2001): (1) *reflective listening* demonstrates that the leaders have heard and understood members; (2) *being empathic, accepting,* and *warm*; (3) *reinforcing* effective interpersonal feedback; (4) communicating at the start of group that discomfort and apprehension about being in groups is normal (i.e., *normalizing behaviors that members may think only they are experiencing*); and (5) *communicating the importance of completing group assignments.*

Measures of Group Cohesion

Most who have written about group psychotherapy have stressed the importance of measuring cohesion. Although several different group cohesion questionnaires have been developed (Kanas, Stewart, Deri, Ketter, & Haney, 1989; MacKenzie, 1983; Treadwell, Lavertue, Kumar, & Veeraraghavan, 2001; Tschuschke et al., 2002), the assessment of group cohesion has not received the research attention it deserves. In the GRIN study, we used the Group Cohesion Questionnaire—Short Version (GCQ-S) because it was brief and easy to score (Kanas et al., 1989; MacKenzie, 1983; Tschuschke et al., 2002).

The 12 items on the GCQ-S are rated on 7-point Likert scales. The measure yields three scores: (1) *Engagement* (5 items, range = 0–30), a positive atmosphere within the group, or cohesiveness; (2) *Conflict* (4 items, range = 0–24), interpersonal friction within the group; and (3) *Avoidance* (3 items, range = 0–18), members not taking personal responsibility for group work. In terms of group cohesion, desirable group characteristics on the GCQ-S would include *high engagement, very low conflict*, and *relatively low avoidance*.

In the GRIN study, all group clients were asked to complete the GCQ-S at their last session (Session 4). After only four sessions, the GRIN study found that the GSC group treatment resulted in high feelings of group cohesiveness and engagement, low levels of interpersonal conflict, and low avoidance of group work (L. C. Sobell et al., 2009). We have postulated that several factors may have contributed to the high cohesiveness: (1) as part of the pregroup preparation, all potential group members were given an introduction that described the group, its benefits, and the expectations of members (Client Handout 5.1); (2) because brief treatments necessitate focusing on specific goals, the development of group processes may have been facilitated because members and leaders knew that the group would meet for only four sessions; (3) group leaders were instructed to reinforce and support the discussion of commonalities and appropriate interactions among members; and (4) the homework exercises and weekly self-monitoring logs of substance use that clients completed outside of the sessions served to focus the group discussions on common themes.

SUMMARY

In this chapter we have focused on three important topics: (1) pregroup planning and preparation, (2) *Music Comes from the Group*, and (3) building group cohesion. Developing group cohesion is essential because it is associated with positive outcomes. Perhaps nothing better captures the importance of group cohesion than the phrase *it is the glue that holds the group together*. As discussed throughout this chapter, there are several ways group leaders can foster the development of cohesion: (1) pregroup planning and preparation, including helping potential members understand their roles and group expectations before joining the group; (2) ensuring that all members have an opportunity to contribute to group discussions; (3) getting members to discuss commonalities and comment on similar experiences they have had; (4) promoting self-disclosure by members; and (5) encouraging members to reinforce other members' behavior changes.

CHAPTER 7

Managing Groups
Structural Issues

> Group therapy is unique in being the only therapy that offers clients the
> opportunity to be of benefit to others. It also encourages role versatility,
> requiring clients to shift between roles of help receivers and help providers.
> —Yalom and Leszcz (2005, p. 13)

This chapter and Chapter 8 are concerned with managing groups, but from different perspectives. This chapter addresses a multitude of structural issues (e.g., composition, attendance, role of cotherapists, breaking eye contact) that are critical for group leaders to understand when conducting group therapy. In contrast, Chapter 8 addresses ways to manage difficult clients in groups.

When comparing group with individual therapy, there are advantages and disadvantages, many of which are structural in nature (Morrison, 2001; Piper & Joyce, 1996; Satterfield, 1994; Stangier, Heidenreich, Peitz, Lauterbach, & Clark, 2003; Yalom & Leszcz, 2005). The major differences between the two formats are listed in Table 7.1. Although managing groups is more com-

---

TABLE 7.1. Advantages and Disadvantages of Group versus Individual Therapy

Advantages

- More clients can be treated in groups, thus reducing costs to clients and payers.
- Groups can provide peer support that cannot be achieved in individual therapy.
- Group members can provide emotional support and reinforcement to each other.
- Groups can help members recognize that others have similar problems.
- Group members can learn from one another (e.g., serve as role models; offer suggestions for changing).

Disadvantages

- More difficult to manage because of simultaneously working with multiple clients, the greater potential for nonparticipation by some members, and the potential problems managing members' behavior (e.g., monopolizing, disruptions).
- Higher dropout rates at entry and over treatment.
- Generally, less client satisfaction with groups.
- Special training and skills needed by therapists to handle complex group dynamics and interactions.
- Attendance issues: missed group sessions cannot be rescheduled; if too many members drop out or miss groups, it can become difficult or impossible to run the group.
- Group members may feel that their confidentiality and/or privacy is less protected.

---

plex, demanding, and challenging than conducting individual therapy, the structure of groups has several important advantages over individual therapy. These advantages, correspondingly, afford members opportunities (e.g., social support) not available in individual therapy.

ASSEMBLING GROUPS

Open Groups

Open groups do not have a fixed number of sessions and, consequently, do not usually have start or stop dates. Space permitting, new members can join at any time. At any given time, because of the nature of open groups, some members will have attended many sessions, others just a few sessions, and others will be new to the group. The mix raises several issues: (1) whenever a new member enters, group rules and expectations must be reviewed; one way to address this is to ask a senior group member to introduce new members to the group and to explain the group rules; (2) session-to-session continuity is harder to maintain; and (3) because of constant member turnover, open groups are not as amenable to structured tasks as are closed groups.

Closed Groups

Closed groups meet for a preset number of sessions with explicit start and stop dates. After the first session, closed groups typically do not add new members. Because all members start simultaneously, to maximize treatment gains closed groups often use structured activities (e.g., homework assignments) and specific topics for different sessions. When the number of group sessions is few, group leaders need to develop group cohesion early (i.e., starting at the first session). A serious issue with closed groups is getting and maintaining a critical mass. We and others have found three things that can help maximize attendance: (1) conduct a pregroup meeting in which potential members are told about the benefits of the group and are given a brochure describing the benefits and the group rules (Client Handout 5.1)—this can be done in a group or individually; (2) stress the importance of attending all group sessions and on time; and (3) very importantly, as a reminder call or e-mail clients the day before each group.

Starting and Stopping Groups on Time

It is imperative to start groups on time even if only a few clients are present rather than waiting for more to arrive because to do otherwise undermines the norm the leaders are trying to instill (Bernard, 1994). Stopping groups on time is similarly important. Although a crisis can occur near the end of group, they are rare and usually can be managed by the leaders after the group. Occasionally, however, members will wait until the end of the group before bringing up a topic. For example, for clients who wait until the last few minutes of group to bring up important, but not crisis-related, issues (e.g., losing a job, getting a C in a class), we recommend that the group leaders respond by saying something like, *"Mary, it sounds like losing your job is an important issue. We want to be able to devote enough time to discussing it in the group, but with only a few minutes left before the group ends, this will be difficult. Do you mind if we discuss it at the start of group next week?"* Most clients will agree with such a request, and one of the group leaders needs to make a note to remember to bring the matter up for discussion at the next session.

Attendance Problems

Attendance problems are not unique to therapy groups. It is common practice, for example, for many professionals and businesses (e.g., doctors, dentists, hairdressers) to call clients or patients to remind them of their appointments. One way to reduce attendance problems is to discuss the importance of attending groups when recruiting potential group members. When clients are constantly late or miss appointments, such behavior can be disruptive and must be addressed. However, it is best to have the group address the issue (i.e., let the "Music Come from the Group") rather than having the group leaders confront members. With clients who repeatedly come late or barge in and disrupt the group, therapists can get the group involved with a comment such as *"This is the third time Mary has been late. I'm wondering how the group can help Mary get to group on time."* Our experience has been that comments from group members are more likely to affect the client's behavior than the therapists' comments.

Missing Groups

When clients fail to attend individual therapy sessions, it is costly for practitioners (i.e., lost time and revenue). However, whereas individual therapy sessions can be rescheduled, if a client misses a group, that group will continue to meet, and there is no way to capture the essence of the group's interactions in a makeup session. Thus, calling clients the day before group sessions can help reduce the number of missed group sessions, and it only takes a few minutes. With clients' permission, a short message about the group can be left on an answering machine or a cell phone. In the GRIN study, the therapists called all group clients the day before their upcoming sessions. It would have required a separate study to evaluate a causal relationship between those calls and attendance, but it is striking that the group members in this study missed far fewer sessions ($n = 25$) than clients in the individual-treatment condition ($n = 210$; L. C. Sobell et al., 2009).

Members Who Rabbit: Leave an Ongoing Group Session

Although it is not common, eventually most group therapists will encounter a group member who walks out of group prematurely, either dramatically or quietly. Although leaving group early should have been discussed as part of the group rules (i.e., members do not leave before the end of the group unless it is an emergency), this will not prevent its occurrence. If a group member attempts to leave or walk out, one of the cotherapists should go after the person to find out why the person left. Group members can walk out for different reasons (e.g., to get attention; because they are angry about what occurred in group). For example, one group member who walked out in the middle of a group session told us that she left because the group discussion brought back vivid memories of an assault she had suffered years earlier. Whatever the reason, one of the cotherapists needs to also leave the group and find out the member's reason for leaving, deal with the situation, and, if appropriate, get the individual to come back to the group. The therapist who remains in the group must trust that if the group member returns, the cotherapist will have the situation under control. The reason that the member chose to leave the group does not necessarily need to be discussed with the rest of the group when the person returns. In addition to not forcing uncomfortable self-disclosures, there is a need to maintain and respect the flow of what has been happening within the ongoing group. Therefore, what has occurred (i.e., the member's leaving) should not be a topic of group discussion unless the leaders feel it is important for group cohesion.

SESSION STRUCTURE: LENGTH AND SIZE

Most outpatient groups meet weekly, and their length typically ranges from 90 to 120 minutes. Although there is no consensus on what constitutes an ideal group size, recommendations vary from 6 to 12 clients with two therapists. One issue for all groups is group size, which can vary from week to week, creating what has been characterized as *feast or famine*. If only a few clients (e.g., one to three) show up for group, our suggestion is to ask them if they want to hold the group. If it is decided that a meaningful group cannot be conducted, then at a minimum we recommend that the group leaders meet with those present for 15–20 minutes to allow them to share how their week went since the previous session and to address any outstanding concerns.

THE ROLE OF COTHERAPISTS/GROUP LEADERS

The consensus among group psychotherapy experts is that using two therapists, called cotherapists, facilitates the conduct of group therapy (Dies, 1994; Yalom & Leszcz, 2005). One therapist typically assumes the active role while the other attends to the nonverbal behaviors of the group members and manages the group activities. In addition, cotherapists can switch roles during the group. There are several advantages to using cotherapists: (1) it is easier to manage and address structured exercises; (2) tasks can be shared—one therapist can manage the clinical tasks (e.g., homework, forms) while the other manages time allotment so all session topics and exercises get discussed; and (3) if one therapist is stuck or uncertain how to proceed, his or her cotherapist can jump in to provide direction.

During all phases of the group, communication between cotherapists is critical (Bieling et al., 2006; Yalom & Leszcz, 2005). For example, during group round-robin discussions one of the cotherapists can monitor the time spent on a topic, while the other therapist is responsible for getting members to participate and share their experiences with each other (see Chapter 5 for specific examples).

Although it is rare for cotherapists to cross-talk or follow one another in a discussion, both need to be communicating, verbally and nonverbally, with each other during sessions (Bernard, 1994). If there is some confusion about what is happening in the group, it is important for cotherapists to check signals with each other. For example, one cotherapist can say to the other, *"Doug, is it okay if we stay on the topic of how to handle relapses a bit longer?"* or *"Doug, help me out. I'm confused about where the group is going with the topic of grief."* Last, although therapists will have different styles and orientations, at times cotherapists may have different ideas about how to proceed. Although this is to be expected, open conflict between cotherapists should be avoided at all costs. If one therapist contradicts the other in front of group members, this can lead the members to question the value of the group and undermine group cohesiveness. The cotherapists can discuss these issues at the postgroup discussion, when group members are absent (reviewed in Morrison, 2001).

Changing Therapists in Open Groups

Because open groups have no start or stop dates, it is conceivable that a cotherapist might leave the group, particularly if one of the cotherapists is a trainee. In such cases, there is a need to be sensitive to the transitioning of both old and new therapists. An important reason for being sensitive to the changing of group therapists is that clients are sharing intimate information with the group, including the therapists. It has been our experience that abrupt changes in group leadership can be disconcerting to clients and should be avoided whenever possible. Ideally, the transition should be gradual, and group members should be informed in advance about when the change in cotherapists will occur. In the open groups that we currently run, we transition our doctoral students as cotherapists every 3 months. Group members are informed in advance about these changes and their rationale, and they also know that one of the two cotherapists will remain, and this provides some stability. In terms of the actual transition, we have found that it works well when we are able to overlap the new therapist with the old therapist for a few weeks. Last, during the transitioning of the old and new cotherapist, it is important to gently work the new cotherapist, especially a trainee, into the flow of the group by having him or her progressively contribute more each session.

SELECTING GROUP MEMBERS: COMPOSITION AND BALANCE

Yalom and Leszcz (2005) have asserted that the fate of a group is related to client selection. Choosing clients who fit common criteria (e.g., divorced clients, trauma victims, problem drinkers) provides a greater potential for bonding between members and for developing cohesion. Moreover, the degree of homogeneity among members is a criterion that has been found to be associated with good group functioning and positive outcomes. In practice, homogeneity allows the leaders to use inherent similarities among group members (e.g., PTSD, substance abuse, relationship issues) to build cohesion by asking them to discuss shared experiences. In seeking harmony in groups, Dies (R. R. Dies, personal communication, February 19, 1996) has suggested applying the principle of Noah's Ark (trying to have at least two members who share a major characteristic). Having at least two members who share a major characteristic is particularly important in some instances (e.g., having more than one woman in a group of male substance abusers).

OTHER SIGNIFICANT GROUP ISSUES

Silence Is Golden

Some therapists, especially new group therapists, have difficulty with silence (Dies, 1994). In this regard, it is important to recognize that silence is a behavior. If no one is speaking for an extended time, something is happening, and the leader might say, *"It's very quiet in here. I'm wondering what is going on?"*

Breaking Eye Contact with Clients

In group therapy, the goal is to have group members mainly talking to other group members and not to the group leaders. When members are new to a group, they often try to maintain eye contact with one of the leaders when speaking. When this occurs, the leader needs to break eye contact with the client. Although this feels awkward and unnatural, our experience has been that when a group leader breaks eye contact, clients will look at another group member and eventually get accustomed to speaking to the *entire* group. Although breaking eye contact is difficult, it is helpful for building group cohesion.

Clients Speak with Their Bodies

People speak with their bodies, such as smiling, nodding, looking away, or crossing one's arms. Nonverbal cues are especially important in groups in which members may be reacting to interactions among members. Although most nonverbal cues relate to body language (e.g., shrugs, smiles, rolling of the eyes), sometimes they will be more obvious (e.g., group members moving their chairs out of the group circle). Group leaders need to be constantly vigilant and acknowledge any significant nonverbal behavior. The following are some examples of how the leaders can bring nonverbal behaviors to the group's attention.

EXAMPLES OF ADDRESSING NONVERBAL RESPONSES

- *"When Mary just talked about her recent divorce, a few of you nodded."* [**Note**: Often when therapists leave their response at this, group members will respond. If there is prolonged silence, the group leader can follow up with, *"What are the nods about?"*]
- *"Several people in the group are smiling. What do the smiles mean?"*
- *"Bill has been sharing some difficult feelings with us, and many of you are looking down. I'm wondering what's happening."*

Clients Who Do Not Complete Their Homework

Another issue related to the group leaders' maintaining control of the group is communicating to members the importance of doing their homework and bringing it to each group session. As discussed in Chapter 3, we (L. C. Sobell et al., 2009) and others (Dies, 1994; Garland & Scott, 2002; Kazantzis et al., 2005) have found that clients will complete homework assignments if they understand their rationale and that the assignments relate to the problems for which they are seeking treatment. Clients can be reminded to bring their homework at the same time the therapist calls them about the group meeting. For clients who regularly fail to bring their homework to the group, therapists can turn the issue over to the group by saying, *"Bill seems to be having trouble completing his homework assignments. What suggestions does the group have for him?"*

Transitioning to a New Topic

As in individual therapy, there will be times when a discussion rambles, gets sidetracked, or continues too long, and this can interfere with addressing other matters. An easy way to address this is to say, *"It sounds like the group has a lot to say on this topic. We have a few more things to cover this session, so let's switch gears and we can come back to this topic later."*

Coming to Groups under the Influence of Substances

Clients who come to groups under the influence of alcohol or illicit drugs not only challenge the group rules but also invite disruptions if they remain in the group. Clients who come to groups under the influence should be reminded that one of the group rules discussed previously was to not use alcohol or drugs on the day of groups. When a client is asked to leave, it is essential that therapists ensure that he or she does not drive home under the influence.

TERMINATION OF GROUPS

The issue of treatment termination is important whether it involves individual or group therapy. Termination involves two critical considerations: addressing unfinished business and helping members plan for what they are going to do after treatment (Dies, 1992). With time-limited groups, the topic of termination should be addressed early in treatment so clients are aware of when the group will end and can plan for what to do if they need additional treatment (Heimberg & Becker, 2002; Yalom & Leszcz, 2005). For many clients, a brief treatment will sufficiently address their needs and result in positive outcomes. For clients seeking additional services, the available alternatives can be discussed with them individually.

Aftercare Calls

As discussed in Chapter 4, part of the GSC treatment model includes having therapists make aftercare phone calls to clients 1 month after the last group or individual session. These calls are intended to be supportive of change while at the same time providing an opportunity for clients to talk about any difficulties they have experienced and to request additional treatment if necessary. In the GRIN study (L. C. Sobell et al., 2009), at the 1-year follow-up, 64% of the substance abusers interviewed said they felt that the aftercare calls were helpful, and 23% said they would have liked more calls.

SUMMARY

This chapter discussed several structural issues involved in the conduct of therapy groups. These issues ranged from differences between open and closed groups to group composition to how to handle members who miss groups, routinely come late, or leave during an ongoing session to breaking eye contact. The complementary roles of cotherapists were addressed. By working together, cotherapists can effectively manage a group while simultaneously observing important features of the developing group process (e.g., nonverbal behaviors). A host of other circumstances that can make conducting therapy groups difficult were discussed, including ways of dealing with those situations. Finally, the major advantages and disadvantages of conducting groups compared with individual therapy are listed in a tabular presentation.

CHAPTER 8

Managing Difficult Clients in Groups

A questionnaire sent by the American Group Psychotherapy Association to practicing group therapists inquired about the critical issues necessary for group therapists to master. Over fifty percent responded, "Working with difficult clients."

—YALOM AND LESZCZ (2005, p. 391)

Group clients bring the full range of their psychopathology to treatment; in addition, the interpersonal, subgroup and group-as-a-whole dynamics that are played out in the group treatment setting result in an enormous range of problematic situations over the course of time.

—BERNARD (1994, p. 156)

Over the years, group therapy experts have commented that therapists can expect to encounter challenging clients and difficult situations when running groups (Bernard, 1994; Bieling et al., 2006; Yalom, 1985). In fact, in their book, Bieling and his colleagues (2006) stated that in their experience "each group a therapist conducts is likely to have at least one client that presents a challenge to group process, to other group members, and to group leaders" (p. 104). Our experience has been similar to that of Bieling and colleagues. It is not uncommon to encounter difficult and challenging clients in groups. Consequently, this chapter addresses ways to manage difficult clients in groups. To help readers picture and remember the clients and behaviors being addressed, we refer to difficult client types with the following shorthand labels: *Silent Sam, Late Laura, Tommie Therapist, Chatty Cathy, Monopolizing Mike, Resistant Roberta*, and *Interrupting Ivan*. Although a discussion of difficult clients is woven into this chapter, Table 8.1 contains specific sample dialogues to give readers a quick reference for ways to respond to such clients in groups.

THINK GROUP: INTERRUPTING CLIENTS FOR THE GREATER GOOD

Interruptions occur frequently in everyday conversations, and as might be expected, they occur during group therapy. However, interruptions during group therapy can interfere with the development of group cohesion. Although isolated interruptions will occur, when clients repeatedly disrupt the group, group leaders need to have the group address the disruptive behaviors, but in a constructive manner.

The following is an example of how group leaders can deal with Chatty Cathy or Monopolizing Mike clients who dominate the group discussion. In such cases, these clients are often

TABLE 8.1. Suggestions for Responding to Difficult Clients in Groups

Silent Sam

With such clients the goal is to find a way to get all members, especially those who are less verbal, to participate in all group sessions.

- *"Mary, we haven't heard from you tonight."*
- *"Mary, I noticed that you haven't said much tonight. How has your week gone?"*
- *"Bill has just shared his frustrations with the group. Mary, I know you've said you felt frustrated in similar situations. What advice can you give Bill?"* [This example directly targets a silent client by asking him or her to offer advice or suggestions to another client.]

Late Laura

Although most clients who come late to groups are aware of their behavior, some fail to understand the effect their behavior has on the group. Having the group respond to such clients is more likely to result in changes (e.g., coming to subsequent groups on time) than is being told they are late by group leaders. The following responses would be used only with clients who are repeatedly late or who miss several group meetings.

- *"This is the third time Mary has been late. What suggestions can the group provide to help her get here on time?"*
- *"I'm wondering how others feel about Mary being late for group several times."* [Although this response is more direct than the first example, open discussion of some issues can increase members' sensitivity to their own behavior, as well as help them understand how their behavior affects the entire group.]

Tommie Therapist

Such clients may have been attending a group for several sessions, or they may have considerable prior therapy experience. At times, such clients' interactions in groups will parallel those of a therapist. Although such advice can sometimes be helpful to group members, on other occasions the advice can be disruptive or too direct.

- *"Bill, your comments have been helpful. Let's see how others view Mary's concerns."*
- *"Bill, that is one way of looking at how Mary can handle the situation. What additional options can others offer Mary?"*

Chatty Cathy and Monopolizing Mike

Such clients dominate group discussions. Group leaders need to find effective ways to interrupt such clients, as they are often unaware of the impact that their behavior has on the group. A strategy that group leaders can use when a Chatty Cathy client is talking is to direct questions to the group as a whole. For example:

- *"Bill, it sounds like a lot has happened with you this week. I am wondering what has happened with other group members."* (The group leader then calls on another member.) *"Mary, how did your week go?"*
- *"Mary, you seem to have had a lot going on this past week. Let's take a look at what's been happening with you for a few more minutes, and then let's see how others have been doing this past week."*

Interrupting Ivan

The behavior of such clients in groups is disruptive, as they frequently interrupt ongoing group discussions.

- *"We seem to be having an active discussion about [insert topic] today, but several members are talking at the same time. I'm wondering how this is affecting the group and what the group thinks we should do."*
- *"I know we all have important things to say, but we need to respect each other and let others finish what they are saying before the next person speaks."*

Resistant Roberta

Clients who feel they are forced or coerced to attend groups (e.g., by a spouse, probation officer, employer) are often not happy and, consequently, participate minimally, if at all.

- *"Bill, as with many people, it appears that you are upset about your probation officer telling you that you have to come to treatment. What suggestions does the group have for Bill?"*
- *"Mary, it sounds like you feel you had no choice in coming to group and you are angry. Who else with similar experiences can share with Mary how they've handled such situations?"*

unaware of the impact their behavior has on the group, and thus group leaders need to find effective ways to interrupt them.

TAKING CONTROL OF THE GROUP

- *"Mary, you seem to have had a lot going on this past week. Let's keep looking at what you're saying for a few more minutes, and then let's see how others have been doing."*
- After a few minutes, the group leader can pull other members in the discussion by saying, *"Mary, clearly a lot has happened with you over the past week. Let's find out how the week has gone for others."* [**Note:** After this comment, the group leader can direct the group discussion by calling on another member.] *"Bill, how did your week go?"*

Over the years, we have found that group leaders may be hesitant to interrupt clients because they are worried about what the other group members will think. In most instances, group leaders need to trust their own feelings as a barometer of what is happening in the group. More often than not, if the group leaders are not comfortable with a member constantly interrupting or talking over other group members, the other members will feel similarly. Moreover, it is unlikely that this is a one-time occurrence (i.e., such clients have been engaging in similar behaviors for some time). With Interrupting Ivans, group leaders need to interrupt them, thank them for sharing their experience, and then pull other members into the discussion. One way to pull other members in when an Interrupting Ivan or a Chatty Cathy is talking is to direct a question to the group as a whole. At such times, it is important for the group leaders to remember to *Think Group*. If the group leaders let one group member go on and on, the rest of the orchestra cannot play well. However, group leaders also must remember to deal with disruptive clients in a way that does not create anger or conflict within the group.

At other times, a group discussion may result in several members speaking at once, and the resulting sound is not music to anyone's ears. On such occasions, the group leaders may find it necessary to call a time-out. In this regard, the group leader acknowledges that there is some confusion and stops the group to figure out what is going on and regroup.

THINK GROUP: BRINGING ORDER TO CHAOS

- *"We seem to be having an active discussion about* [**insert topic**] *today. There are a lot of folks talking at once. I'm wondering how the interruptions are affecting the group, and what the group thinks we should do?"*
- If several members are talking at once, the leader could say, *"I know we all have important things to say, but we need to respect each other and let others finish before the next person speaks."*

BALANCING VOICES IN THE GROUP

A major goal for group leaders when conducting groups is having all clients participate regularly. With Silent Sam clients it is important for group leaders to make active and continuous efforts to get them involved in the group. Such efforts are important for developing group cohesion. To do this, the group leaders must orchestrate opportunities to prompt reluctant or shy group members to participate. For example, the group leader could say, *"Mary, we haven't heard from you tonight"* or *"Mary, you have been quiet tonight. How did your week go?"* A good way of getting silent clients to participate is for the group leaders to recognize commonalities and steer the discussion in that direction: *"Bill has just shared his frustrations with the group. Mary, I know you've told us you have felt frustrated in similar situations. What advice can you give Bill?"* Not all group members have to speak at length on every topic, but it is desirable to have a balance of voices in the group.

Time management is an issue that makes balancing voices very important, particularly for time-limited groups (Heimberg & Becker, 2002; MacKenzie, 1996). A good example is handling clients known as *storytellers*. Such members, if left unmanaged, can derail a group with long, rambling stories. In time-limited groups, group leaders need to be vigilant in attending to group processes, and when the group gets sidetracked, one of the group leaders needs to bring the group back on topic.

Sometimes the issue of balancing voices involves the roles clients take on rather than the amount of time that they speak, such as with a Tommie Therapist client. Such clients may have been attending a group for several sessions, or they may have considerable prior therapy experience. Whatever the reason, at times they attempt to take on the role of therapist. On occasion, this can be very helpful. For example, in an open group, a senior group member can explain group rules to new members and help ease their transition into the group. Such clients, however, can also be disruptive if they start to give advice freely or provide their opinions as if they were trained therapists. In such cases, a group leader could say, *"Bill, that is one way of looking at how Mary can handle the situation. What additional options can others think of for Mary?"*

Another issue relates to group members who feel they are forced or coerced to attend groups (e.g., by a spouse, probation officer, employer). Resistant Roberta clients are often not happy, and consequently they participate minimally, if at all, in groups. Like clients who are late, clients who are forced to come to group are best managed by the leaders using the group as the agent of change. With such clients, the group leader can ask the group to comment about a member's behavior. For example, the group leader could say, *"Bill, as with many people, it appears that you are upset about your probation officer telling you that you have to come to treatment. What suggestions does the group have for Bill?"* In such situations, other group members are likely to share how they have coped with circumstances in which they have had little choice. Such responses can also be directly encouraged by the leader saying, *"Mary, it sounds like you feel you had no choice in coming to group, and you are angry. Who else with similar experiences can share with Mary how they've handled such situations?"* As discussed in Chapter 6, having the "Music Come from the Group" typically will be more effective than having the group leaders isolate or lecture a group member.

MANAGING CONFLICT AND CALLING TIME-OUTS

Yalom and Leszcz (2005) state that, "To some degree, certain tensions are always present in every therapy group" (p. 169). In fact, most group psychotherapy experts acknowledge that some degree of conflict in groups is normal and unavoidable. Such is not at all surprising when we remember that groups consist of multiple clients with different personalities. When conflicts do arise, however, cotherapists must recognize them and manage them to a successful resolution. Many clients, particularly in a group setting, will feel uncomfortable with conflict or anger expressed in a group. At such times, one of the group leaders needs to address the discomfort with the group as a whole. For example, the group leader might say, *"There is a lot going on right now, some of which feels a bit uncomfortable. Let's talk some about what we think this is about."* Alternately, the group leaders can ask specific clients to comment: *"Bill and Mary, a lot has been happening in group tonight, and you both look a bit uncomfortable. What do you think is going on?"* Sometimes when a group leader interrupts the group's discussion to reflect back what is happening, it can have a secondary gain by allowing group members who are upset to calm down.

Therapists Should Use Their Feelings as a Barometer

Group leaders need to use their own feelings as a barometer of what is happening *affectively* in the group (Dies, 1994). For example, if the group leaders are reacting to the member-to-member interactions, then it is likely that other members are having similar feelings. Although some conflict in groups is to be expected, the best way to manage group conflict is for the group leaders to throw it back to the group. There are times, however, when dealing with the conflict might not be immediately productive, and on these occasions, time-outs can be helpful.

Time-outs are typically called in relation to very strong emotional reactions the group has had to what a member has said. In such cases, the group leader calls a time-out by saying, *"Okay, let's take a time-out. It seems like a lot is going on in group right now. Let's all step back a minute and process what just happened."* On rare occasions, leaders may have to get the group's attention by calling a time-out similar to that of a basketball coach by forming their hands into a *"T."* During the time-out the group leaders need to focus the discussion on the group's affective response to the situation, rather than the topic being discussed. For example, suppose the topic was domestic violence, and one member asserted that his partner deserved to be hit. This could easily escalate as other members react strongly and negatively to what the one member said. Likewise, there may be times when members are so upset that the most prudent thing to do is to let them calm down. Here a group leader might say, *"Right now things seem very emotional. I think it might be best for us to come back and revisit this topic next week when we've all had some time to reflect on what happened in group today."*

In summary, when calling a time-out or when responding to an interruption, it is important to focus on the *affect* that members are experiencing rather than the issue at hand. In the end, the group leaders need to remember to be supportive of all group members for their contribution to the group. In this regard, the group leader could say, *"Sometimes difficult issues get raised in groups. However, we can learn from different perspectives and by addressing difficult issues in a reasoned, calm manner as we have done here."* Such an approach also allows the disruptive member or members to observe appropriate ways to discuss sensitive topics.

SELF-DISCLOSURE

Self-Disclosure by Clients

Although there may be disagreement about what to disclose, experts in group psychotherapy such as Yalom and Leszcz (2005) and Dies (1992) agree that *"self-disclosure is absolutely essential in the group therapeutic process"* (Yalom & Leszcz, 2005, p. 130, original emphasis). However, if a client discloses embarrassing or sensitive information and the group is not supportive or no one responds, this can affect whether members self-disclose in the future or even return to the next group session. Members may not respond because they do not know what to say or because they feel very uncomfortable about what was disclosed. In either case, the group leaders need to reflect what happened and reinforce self-disclosure. For example, *"Mary just told us about a very personal situation in her life, and no one said anything."* When group leaders say something along these lines, it gives those in the group permission to comment. Another way group leaders can attempt to get members responding if one member self-discloses and no one responds is to say, *"I am wondering how we can offer Mary support with respect to what she has told us?"* In terms of reinforcing a client's self-disclosure in group, one of the group leaders might say, *"I notice that Mary has taken a big step by revealing some very personal things about herself. This must have been difficult. How do others in group feel about what Mary just said?"* Finally, the group can also be prompted to use self-disclosure as a starting point for sharing: *"Bill took a big risk in sharing what happened to him over the past week. Who else can relate to what happened to Bill?"*

Inappropriate Client Self-Disclosure

Another issue for consideration relates to members bringing up topics (e.g., abuse) that are not deemed appropriate for the group discussion. Frequently, such issues relate to only one client and are not appropriate for the group unless the entire group is dealing with similar issues (e.g., a PTSD group). In addition, when inappropriate topics are disclosed in group, they can negatively affect group cohesion. For example, when trauma survivors disclose details of their traumatic incident, it can lead to concern about how the other group members perceive them and to their decompensating. In addition, if the group members respond with little or no empathy or if they sound judgmental, it can add to the blame or guilt that these clients (i.e., trauma survivors) might be experiencing.

The introduction of inappropriate topics is usually easy to recognize (e.g., other members will look down and/or there is total silence). When group leaders recognize that a topic is not appropriate for the rest of the group, they can say, *"Mary, although it sounds like that is an important issue for you, often such concerns are better handled in individual therapy. Let me follow up with you after the group."* There are, of course, several kinds of issues that might be inappropriate for groups. More often than not, such issues do not relate to what brought the group members into treatment (e.g., upcoming political elections; political views; discussing how one feels about gays and lesbians in a smoking cessation group). In the end, decisions about the appropriateness of topics rest with the judgment of the group leaders.

Self-Disclosure by Therapists

In group therapy, the phrase *self-disclosure by therapists* has a different meaning from the way that phrase would be used in individual therapy (Dies, 1994). In individual therapy, self-disclosure usually refers to therapists' revealing information about themselves (e.g., *"I've been divorced twice"* or *"I've smoked marijuana once, too"*). In contrast, self-disclosures by cotherapists in a group typically are expressions of *here-and-now feelings* about what is happening in the group. For example, a group leader might say, *"I'm feeling uncomfortable with what has just happened. Who else is feeling that way?"* Of course, self-disclosures by group leaders could involve revealing personal information to the group. However, in such cases the disclosure should have a specific intent or therapeutic rationale, as would be the case in individual therapy.

Therapist self-disclosure of feelings about the group can provide a good way of dealing with dilemmas around difficult topics and issues, especially when the leaders are having trouble gauging the group's reaction. Following are some examples of how this can be accomplished.

EXAMPLES OF THERAPIST SELF-DISCLOSURES RELATED TO FEELINGS ABOUT THE GROUP

- *"It feels like there is some tension in the room after what just happened. I wonder how others are feeling?"*
- *"I get the feeling that everyone would like to say more about the situation, but many of you seem to be a bit anxious talking about* **[insert sensitive topic]**.*"*
- *"What does the group think is happening?"*
- *"Mary, we can't imagine what that must have been like for you. Can you share how you are feeling right now with the group?"*
- *"It sounds as if everyone is feeling a bit anxious."*

PERSONALIZING PROBLEMS USING AFFECT

Another key way of encouraging members to become more involved in the group is to personalize problems and get members to discuss their feelings (Dies, 1994). Following are a few examples of how therapists can encourage such discussion while centering on affect.

EXAMPLES OF GETTING MEMBERS TO PERSONALIZE PROBLEMS USING AFFECT

- *"Mary, how would it feel to be in that situation?"*
- *"Bill, that sounds like it has been difficult for you. Who else has had similar experiences?"*
- *"How have others felt when similar things have happened to them?"*
- *"How would you feel if that were to happen to you?"*
- *"How does that relate to why you are here?"*

SUMMARY

In several chapters throughout this book, including the present one, we have discussed skills therapists need to effectively conduct and manage groups. These skills include (1) building cohesion by looking for commonalities among members; (2) using reflective listening; (3) ensuring that all group members participate regularly; (4) managing multiple clients at one time; (5) managing resistance and dealing with conflict; (6) turning difficult situations into learning opportunities for group members; and (7) most important, letting the "music come from the group."

CHAPTER 9

The Way Ahead

Savings from transitioning to the most cost-effective treatment modality may free resources that could be reinvested to improve access to substance abuse treatment for a larger number of individuals in need of such treatment.
—MOJTABAI AND ZIVIN (2003, p. 233)

Knowledge of individual psychopathology and clinical interventions is necessary but not sufficient to become a skilled group therapist.
—MARKUS AND KING (2003, p. 203)

Health and mental health care costs have risen steadily over the past decade (Cummings, O'Donohue, & Ferguson, 2002; Orszag, 2008). Rising costs put increased pressure on health and mental health providers, insurance companies, policy makers, and politicians to monitor and provide information about the efficacy and efficiency of services provided. Part and parcel of such scrutiny is an increased concern for accountability.

For all areas of health and mental health, central planning issues concern cost containment and how to allocate limited resources. Cost-effectiveness is the intersection of efficacy and efficiency. From this perspective, evidence-based treatments are the starting but not the end point of cost containment considerations. For example, cost-effectiveness can be expected to play a major role in funding decisions when comparing two or more equally effective treatments. In practice, this means that for more expensive or resource-intensive treatments to be selected, they must produce outcomes much better than less costly treatments in order to justify the additional costs. This suggests that group therapy will increasingly be the treatment of choice except when there is evidence of superior outcomes with individual treatment. Presently, demonstrations of such superiority are lacking.

PUTTING COST-EFFECTIVE TREATMENTS INTO PRACTICE

There is considerable evidence that brief treatments should, in most cases, be the first treatment of choice for those with SUDs. Studies evaluating different treatment formats and lengths have favored briefer, less resource-intensive treatments and services, whether they have compared outpatient with inpatient treatment, outpatient detoxification with inpatient detoxification, or brief treatments with a few minutes of physician advice (Feldman, Pattison, Sobell, Graham, & Sobell, 1975; Fleming et al., 1997; French, 2000; Heather, 1989; Holder, Longabaugh, Miller, & Rubonis, 1991; Longabaugh et al., 1983). In addition, although intensive treatments for SUDS have not been shown to be any more effective than less intensive treatments, they are more costly (Mojtabai & Zivin, 2003). In this regard, although some individuals in brief treatments will not improve and will need additional services, such concerns can be addressed using a stepped-care model of treatment similar to that used in the medical field (Davison, 2000; M. B. Sobell & Sobell, 2000).

Stepped-Care Treatment Model

As shown in Figure 9.1, when using a stepped-care model the first intervention is evidence-based, usually the least intensive and intrusive, and has consumer appeal and a reasonable chance of success. If the first treatment produces satisfactory results, monitoring and follow-up visits may be all that are necessary. If the intervention does not produce positive results, treatment can be "stepped up" by extending the same treatment (i.e., more sessions) or implementing a different and perhaps more intensive intervention (e.g., pharmacotherapy for smokers in behavioral treatment that is not currently effective). Using a stepped-care model, decisions about further treatment are based on a person's response to previous treatments. In this way, only those needing services that are more intensive receive the more costly treatments.

The substance abuse field, albeit slowly, has been moving in the direction of less intensive treatments. For example, in the early 1980s the vast majority of alcohol and drug treatment programs were inpatient or residential, but today such treatment programs are in the minority (Substance Abuse and Mental Health Administration, 2003; Swift & Miller, 1997). As cost containment continues, it can be expected that services will be evidence-based and cost-effective. In this regard, the time-limited group treatment described in this book is evidence-based, consistent with a stepped-care model of service delivery, and would be a good first treatment of choice for many individuals with SUDs.

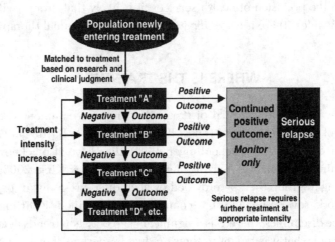

FIGURE 9.1. Stepped-care model of treatment. From M. B. Sobell and Sobell (1993b, p. 150). Copyright 1993 by Sage Publications, Inc. Adapted by permission.

ARE GROUPS COST-EFFECTIVE?

As discussed in Chapter 1, the number of studies that have evaluated the cost-effectiveness (i.e., presented cost and time figures) of group therapy is limited. However, as seen in the following example, it is easy to make a prima facie case that groups have a cost-effectiveness edge over individual therapy.

COST EFFECTIVENESS OF GROUP VERSUS INDIVIDUAL THERAPY

Example: Eight clients seen for six weekly sessions

- **Individual therapy**: 1-hour session conducted by 1 therapist
- **Group therapy**: 2-hour sessions conducted by 2 therapists
- **Therapist time for individual sessions: 48 hours** [8 different clients x 6 sessions each (1 hour per week) x 1 therapist]
- **Therapist time for group sessions: 24 hours** [6 group sessions (with 8 clients per group) x 2 hours per group session x 2 therapists]

The preceding example results in a 50% savings of therapist time for group therapy versus individual therapy. Moreover, the efficiency advantage for all groups is greater with more clients per group. Consider the preceding example with 10 rather than 8 clients. The individual therapist time would be 60 hours, whereas the group therapist time for 10 clients (i.e., 6 sessions × 2 hours per group session × 2 therapists) would still be 24 hours, which is a 60% savings in therapist time. In fact, in the randomized controlled trial of group versus individual GSC treatment described earlier in this book, a similar analysis found that group therapy produced a savings of 41.4% in the therapist's time (L. C. Sobell et al., 2009). In addition, if a member misses a group, the group session still takes place. However, when clients fail to attend individual sessions, therapists cannot use this time to see other clients. Thus, even in the absence of studies of cost-effectiveness, there is a significant advantage to group therapy. As cost containment continues to be a priority in the provision of health services, it is likely that groups will be favored over individual therapy unless there is a specific justification for individual therapy.

WHERE IS THE TRAINING?

Over the years, as experts in the field of group therapy have commented on the challenges and complexities of conducting groups (Dies, 1980; Fuhriman & Burlingame, 2001; Markus & King, 2003; Piper & Joyce, 1996; Scheidlinger, 1994), they have also acknowledged the need for adequate training (Fuhriman & Burlingame, 2001; Markus & King, 2003; Thorn, 2004). In a survey of training in group therapy provided by accredited programs in psychiatry, psychology, and social work, several notable shortcomings were identified (Fuhriman & Burlingame, 2001). For all three disciplines, there was a significant gap between trends occurring in the field of group therapy and what was taught in their graduate programs. For example, although 83% of psychologists surveyed conduct group psychotherapy, only 21% had been required to take a group therapy course or practicum as part of their training.

If, as predicted, the prevalence of group therapy continues to increase over the next several years, a serious priority will be to ensure that there are competently trained therapists to conduct groups. Because of the challenges and complexities of conducting group therapy, training needs to include more than didactic seminars (Markus & King, 2003). Rather, there should be a major focus on group therapy as a part of professional training, analogous to how training is provided for individual therapy.

GROUP THERAPY: THE WAVE OF THE FUTURE

For 20 years, Norcross and colleagues have been conducting Delphi polls using a panel of experts to predict trends in psychotherapy. In the most recent survey (Norcross, Hedges, & Prochaska, 2002), experts predicted that four therapy formats would increase, two of which are group and short-term therapy. If one were to speculate as to why these two formats were included, it would likely relate to their economic advantage over long-term therapy formats that were judged to be on the decline. It also might reflect an increasing recognition that change often occurs early in treatment.

Group Therapy in the Health Care System of the Future

As discussed in Chapter 1, the literature provides evidence of equal effectiveness and lower costs for groups compared with individual therapy. This is consistent with the outcome of the GRIN study. The similar outcomes for group and individual therapy will make it difficult for practitioners to ignore groups as an effective and cost-efficient treatment modality in the future.

Based on what we have presented in this book, the following comments are offered with respect to group therapy and its place in our future health care system.

- Pressures to contain rising health care costs will continue to increase, with an emphasis on providing less costly, evidence-based services, including group therapy.
- Although health care cost containment is necessary, it must not jeopardize quality of care.
- Group therapy is complex and challenging, and group therapists need to be adequately trained.
- Most graduate training programs need to change their curricula to ensure that practitioners are competently trained to provide group therapy.
- More research is needed on how to make groups more acceptable to clients.
- Treatment services should be provided consistent with a stepped-care treatment model in order to maximize efficiency without sacrificing individualized care.

SUMMARY

In this final chapter, we suggested that time-limited group therapy is a cost-effective intervention in a stepped-care model of treatment. Throughout this book we have made the case, as have other group therapy experts, that conducting group therapy is complex and challenging.

To this end, however, adequate training in how to effectively conduct and manage the dynamics of interpersonal interactions in groups is lacking at many levels. Nevertheless, as pressure for health care cost containment continues to mount, time-limited group therapy will be viewed as cost-effective in general and an approach particularly well suited for helping individuals whose health and mental health problems are not severe. In summary, as the popularity of group therapy has grown over the past decade, a major challenge will be to ensure that there are competently trained practitioners to conduct such groups.

APPENDICES

AUDIT Questionnaire

---

1 Standard Drink is Equal to

 One 12 oz. can/bottle of beer   One 5 oz. glass of regular (12%) wine   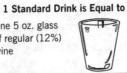 1½ oz. of hard liquor (e.g., rum, vodka, whiskey)   1 mixed or straight drink with 1½ oz. hard liquor

---

These questions refer to your use of alcohol. Please circle the answer that is correct for you.

1. How often do you have a drink containing alcohol?

0	1	2	3	4
never	monthly or less	2 to 4 times/month	2 to 3 times/week	4 or more times/week

2. How many drinks containing alcohol do you have on a typical day when you are drinking?

0	0	1	2	3	4
none	1 or 2	3 or 4	5 or 6	7 to 9	10 or more

3. How often do you have six or more drinks on one occasion?

0	1	2	3	4
never	less than monthly	monthly	weekly	daily or almost daily

4. How often during the last year have you found that you were not able to stop drinking once you had started?

0	1	2	3	4
never	less than monthly	monthly	weekly	daily or almost daily

5. How often during the last year have you failed to do what was normally expected from you because of drinking?

0	1	2	3	4
never	less than monthly	monthly	weekly	daily or almost daily

6. How often during the last year have you needed a first drink in the morning to get yourself going after a heavy drinking session?

0	1	2	3	4
never	less than monthly	monthly	weekly	daily or almost daily

7. How often during the last year have you had a feeling of guilt or remorse after drinking?

0	1	2	3	4
never	less than monthly	monthly	weekly	daily or almost daily

8. How often during the last year have you been unable to remember what happened the night before because you had been drinking?

0	1	2	3	4
never	less than monthly	monthly	weekly	daily or almost daily

9. Have you or someone else been injured as a result of your drinking?

0	2	4
no	yes, but not in the last year	yes, during the last year

10. Has a relative or friend or a doctor or other health worker been concerned about your drinking or suggested you cut down?

0	2	4
no	yes, but not in the last year	yes, during the last year

AUDIT Score: _____

(cont.)

From Saunders, J. B., Aasland, O. G., Babor, T. F., De La Fuente, J. R., & Grant, M. (1993). Development of the Alcohol Use Disorders Identification Test (AUDIT): WHO collaborative project on early detection of persons with harmful alcohol consumption—II. *Addiction, 88*, 791–804. The AUDIT is copyrighted by Wiley-Blackwell but can be reproduced without permission.

AUDIT SCORING KEY

- The Alcohol Use Disorders Identification Test (AUDIT) was developed by the World Health Organization to evaluate a person's use of alcohol and the extent to which drinking is a problem.
- The AUDIT contains 10 questions. Most questions relate to the past year while a few ask about lifetime use.
- Questions are scored from 0 to 4. Scores can range from 0 to 40.
- Higher scores typically reflect problems that are more serious.
- If a person's score is 8 or greater, it is suggestive of an alcohol problem.
- The AUDIT is available in several languages and can be freely used as it is in the public domain.

SCORES RELATED TO SEVERITY OF ALCOHOL USE

Score	Degree of Alcohol Problem Severity
0	None
1–7	Low
8–16	Moderate
17–25	High
26–40	Very High

Drug Use Questionnaire (DAST-10)

The following questions concern information about your potential involvement with drugs excluding alcohol and tobacco during the past 12 months. Carefully read each statement and decide if your answer is "No" or "Yes." Then fill in the appropriate box beside the question.

When the words "drug abuse" are used, they mean the use of prescribed or over-the-counter drugs in excess of the directions and any nonmedical use of drugs. The various classes of drugs may include cannabis (e.g., marijuana, hash), solvents, tranquilizers (e.g., Valium), barbiturates, cocaine, stimulants (e.g., speed), hallucinogens (e.g., LSD), or narcotics (e.g., heroin). Remember that the questions do not include alcohol or tobacco.

Please answer every question. If you have difficulty with a statement, then choose the response that is mostly right.

These questions refer to the past 12 months: No   Yes

1. Have you used drugs other than those required for medical reasons?   _____   _____

2. Do you abuse more than one drug at a time?   _____   _____

3. Are you always able to stop using drugs when you want to?   _____   _____

4. Have you had "blackouts" or "flashbacks" as a result of drug use?   _____   _____

5. Do you ever feel bad or guilty about your drug use?   _____   _____

6. Does your spouse (or parents) ever complain about your involvement   _____   _____
   with drugs?

7. Have you neglected your family because of your use of drugs?   _____   _____

8. Have you engaged in illegal activities in order to obtain drugs?   _____   _____

9. Have you ever experienced withdrawal symptoms (felt sick) when you   _____   _____
   stopped taking drugs?

10. Have you had medical problems as a result of your drug use (e.g., memory   _____   _____
    loss, hepatitis, convulsions, bleeding, etc.)?

(cont.)

Skinner, H. A. (1982). The Drug Abuse Screening Test. *Addictive Behaviors, 7,* 363–371. The DAST-10 is in the public domain and can be freely copied.

DAST-10 SCORING KEY

SCORING: For every **"Yes"** answer to Questions 1–2 and 4–10 score 1 point, and for Question 3 score 1 point for a **"No"** answer.

SCORE	DEGREE OF PROBLEM RELATED TO DRUG ABUSE
0	No Problem Reported
1–2	Low Problem Level
3–5	Moderate Problem Level
6–8	Substantial Problem Level
9–10	Severe Problem Level

Drug Use History Questionnaire

DRUG CATEGORY (Includes nonmedical drug use) **Note:** Use card sort with drug category names to first determine which drugs have ever been used, then ask for information for the drugs ever used	Ever Used Circle Yes or No[a]	Total Years Used[b]	Intravenous Drug Use NA = Not Applicable	Year Last Used (e.g., 1998)	Frequency of Use Past 6 Months[c]
ALCOHOL	No Yes		NA		
CANNABIS: Marijuana, hashish, hash oil	No Yes		NA		
STIMULANTS: Cocaine, crack	No Yes		No Yes		
STIMULANTS: Methamphetamine—speed, ice, crank	No Yes		No Yes		
AMPHETAMINES/OTHER STIMULANTS: Ritalin, Benzedrine, Dexedrine	No Yes		NA		
BENZODIAZEPINES/ TRANQUILIZERS: Valium, Librium, Xanax, Diazepam, Roofies	No Yes		NA		
SEDATIVES/HYPNOTICS/ BARBITURATES: Amytal, Seconal, Dalmane, Quaalude, Phenobarbital	No Yes		NA		
HEROIN	No Yes		No Yes		
STREET OR ILLICIT METHADONE	No Yes		NA		
OTHER OPIOIDS: Tylenol #2 & #3, 282's, 292's, Percodan, Percocet, Opium, Morphine, Demerol, Dilaudid	No Yes		NA		
HALLUCINOGENS: LSD, PCP, STP, MDA, DAT, mescaline, peyote, mushrooms, ecstasy (MDMA), nitrous oxide	No Yes		NA		
INHALANTS: Glue, gasoline, aerosols, paint thinner, poppers, rush, locker room	No Yes		NA		
[a]**If EVER USED is NO** for any given line, the **remainder of the line should be left blank.**	[b]**Infrequent Use** (= 2 x/year) **or Brief Experimental Use** (< 3 months lifetime use) = **write 87**		[c]**Frequency Codes:** **0** = no use **4** = 1x/wk. **1** = < 1x/mo. **5** = 2 to 3x/wk. **2** = 1x/mo. **6** = 4 to 6x/wk. **3** = 2 to 3x/mo. **7** = daily		

From Sobell, L. C., Kwan, E., & Sobell, M. B. (1995). The reliability of a Drug History Questionnaire (DHQ). *Addictive Behaviors, 20*, 233–241. Copyright 1995, with permission from Elsevier.

Brief Situational Confidence Questionnaire (BSCQ)

Listed below are eight types of situations in which some people experience an alcohol or drug problem. The questions are to be answered in relation to your alcohol or primary drug problem.

Imagine yourself as you are **right now** in each of the following types of situations. Indicate on the scale provided how confident you are **right now** that you would be able to resist drinking heavily or resist the urge to use your primary drug in each situation by placing an "**X**" along the line, from **0% "Not At All Confident"** to **100% "Totally Confident,"** as in the example below.

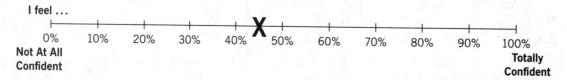

Right now I would be able to resist the urge to drink heavily or resist the urge to use my primary drug in situations involving . . .

1. **UNPLEASANT EMOTIONS** (e.g., If I were depressed about things in general; If everything was going badly for me).

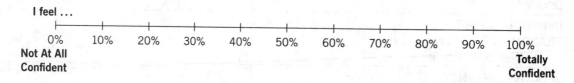

2. **PHYSICAL DISCOMFORT** (e.g., If I would have trouble sleeping; If I felt jumpy and physically tense).

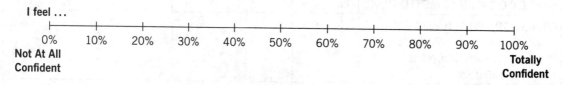

3. **PLEASANT EMOTIONS** (e.g., If something good would happen and I would feel like celebrating; if everything was going well).

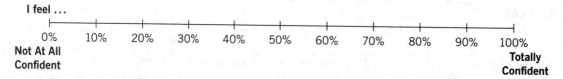

(cont.)

Right now I would be able to resist the urge to drink heavily or resist the urge to use my primary drug in situations involving ...

4. **TESTING CONTROL OVER MY USE OF ALCOHOL or DRUGS** (e.g., If I would start to believe that alcohol or drugs were no longer a problem for me; If I would feel confident that I could handle drugs or several drinks).

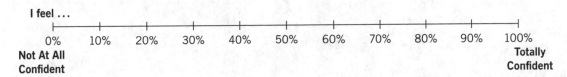

5. **URGES AND TEMPTATIONS** (e.g., If I suddenly had an urge to drink or use drugs; If I were in a situation where I had often used drugs or drank heavily; If I began to think of how good a rush or high had felt).

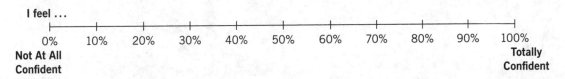

6. **CONFLICT WITH OTHERS** (e.g., If I had an argument with a friend; If I were not getting along well with others at work).

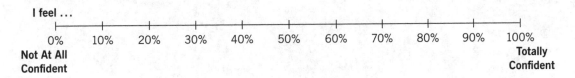

7. **SOCIAL PRESSURE TO USE** (e.g., If someone would pressure me to "be a good sport" and drink or use drugs with them; If I would be invited to someone's home and they would offer me a drink or drugs).

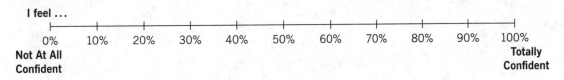

8. **PLEASANT TIMES WITH OTHERS** (e.g., If I wanted to celebrate with a friend; If I would be enjoying myself at a party and wanted to feel even better).

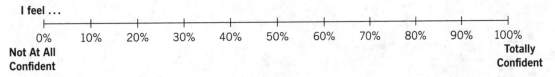

References

Abrams, D. B., & Wilson, G. T. (1979). Effects of alcohol on social anxiety in women: Cognitive versus physiological processes. *Journal of Abnormal Psychology, 88*(2), 161–173.

Addis, M. E., & Jacobson, N. S. (2000). A closer look at the treatment rationale and homework compliance in cognitive-behavioral therapy for depression. *Cognitive Therapy and Research, 24*(3), 313–326.

Agrawal, S., Sobell, M. B., & Sobell, L. C. (2008). The Timeline Followback: A scientifically and clinically useful tool for assessing substance use. In R. F. Belli, F. P. Stafford, & D. F. Alwin (Eds.), *Calendar and time diary methods in life course research* (pp. 57–68). Beverly Hills, CA: Sage.

Allsop, S. (2007). What is this thing called motivational interviewing? *Addiction, 102*(3), 343–345.

Andréasson, S., Hansagi, H., & Oesterlund, B. (2002). Short-term treatment for alcohol-related problems: Four-session guided self-change versus one session of advice—A randomized controlled trial. *Alcohol, 28*(1), 57–62.

Annis, H. M. (Ed.). (1986). *A relapse prevention model for the treatment of alcoholics.* New York: Pergamon Press.

Annis, H. M., & Davis, C. S. (1988). Assessment of expectancies. In D. M. Donovan & G. A. Marlatt (Eds.), *Assessment of addictive behaviors* (pp. 84–111). New York: Guilford Press.

Apodaca, T. R., & Longabaugh, R. (2009). Mechanisms of change in motivational interviewing: A review and preliminary evaluation of the evidence. *Addiction, 104*(5), 705–715.

Ayala, H. E., Echeverría, L., Sobell, M., & Sobell, L. (1997). Auto control dirigido: Intervenciones breves para bebedores problema en Mexico. *Revista Mexicana de Psicología, 14*(2), 113–127.

Ayala, H. E., Echeverría, L., Sobell, M. B., & Sobell, L. C. (1998). Una alternativa de intervencin breve y temprana parabebedores problema en México [An early and brief intervention alternative for problem drinkers in Mexico]. *Acta Comportamentalia, 6,* 71–93.

Ayala-Velazquez, H., Cardenas, C., Echeverria, L., & Gutierrez, M. (1995). Initial results of an autocontrol program for problem alcoholics in Mexico. *Salud Mental, 18*(4), 18–24.

Babor, T. F., Higgins-Biddle, J. C., Dauser, D., Burleson, J. A., Zarkin, G. A., & Bray, J. (2006). Brief interventions for at-risk drinking: Patient outcomes and cost-effectiveness in managed care organizations. *Alcohol and Alcoholism, 41*(6), 624–631.

Babor, T. F., Steinberg, K., Anton, R., & Del Boca, F. (2000). Talk is cheap: Measuring drinking outcomes in clinical trials. *Journal of Studies on Alcohol, 61*(1), 55–63.

Bandura, A. (1977). Self-efficacy: Toward a unifying theory of behavioral change. *Psychological Review, 84,* 191–215.

Bandura, A. (1986). *Social foundations of thought and action: A social cognitive theory*. Englewood Cliffs, NJ: Prentice-Hall.

Barlow, S. H., Burlingame, G. M., Nebeker, R. S., & Anderson, E. (2000). Meta-analysis of medical self-help groups. *International Journal of Group Psychotherapy, 50*(1), 53–69.

Baumeister, R. F. (1994). The crystallization of discontent in the process of major life change. In T. F. Heatherton & J. L. Weinberger (Eds.), *Can personality change?* (pp. 281–297). Washington, DC: American Psychological Association.

Beal, D. J., Cohen, R. R., Burke, M. J., & McLendon, C. L. (2003). Cohesion and performance in groups: A meta-analytic clarification of construct relations. *Journal of Applied Psychology, 88*(6), 989–1004.

Bernard, H. S. (1994). Difficult patients and challenging situations. In H. S. Bernard & K. R. MacKenzie (Eds.), *Basics of group psychotherapy* (pp. 123–156). New York: Guilford Press.

Bernard, H. S., & MacKenzie, K. R. (Eds.). (1994). *Basics of group psychotherapy*. New York: Guilford Press.

Berridge, V. (1999). Histories of harm reduction: Illicit drugs, tobacco, and nicotine. *Substance Use and Misuse, 34*(1), 35–47.

Bieling, P. J., McCabe, R. E., & Antony, M. M. (2006). *Cognitive-behavioral therapy in groups*. New York: Guilford Press.

Brandsma, J. M., & Pattison, E. M. (1985). The outcome of group psychotherapy alcoholics: An empirical review. *American Journal of Drug and Alcohol Abuse, 11*, 151–162.

Breslin, C., Li, S., Sdao-Jarvie, K., Tupker, E., & Ittig-Deland, V. (2002). Brief treatment for young substance abusers: A pilot study in an addiction treatment setting. *Psychology of Addictive Behaviors, 16*(1), 10–16.

Breslin, F. C., Sobell, L. C., Sobell, M. B., & Agrawal, S. (2000). A comparison of a brief and long version of the Situational Confidence Questionnaire. *Behaviour Research and Therapy, 38*(12), 1211–1220.

Breslin, F. C., Sobell, M. B., Sobell, L. C., Buchan, G., & Cunningham, J. A. (1997). Toward a stepped care approach to treating problem drinkers: The predictive utility of within-treatment variables and therapist prognostic ratings. *Addiction, 92*(11), 1479–1489.

Breslin, F. C., Sobell, M. B., Sobell, L. C., Cunningham, J. A., Sdao-Jarvie, K., & Borsoi, D. (1998). Problem-drinkers: Evaluation of stepped-care approach. *Journal of Substance Abuse, 10*(3), 217–232.

Britt, E., Blampied, N. M., & Hudson, S. M. (2003). Motivational interviewing: A review. *Australian Psychologist, 38*(3), 193–201.

Budman, S. H., Demby, A., Redondo, J. P., Hannan, M., Feldstein, M., Ring, J., et al. (1988). Comparative outcome in time-limited individual and group psychotherapy. *International Journal of Group Psychotherapy, 38*, 63–86.

Burke, B. L., Arkowitz, H., & Menchola, M. (2003). The efficacy of motivational interviewing: A meta-analysis of controlled clinical trials. *Journal of Consulting and Clinical Psychology, 71*(5), 843–861.

Burlingame, G. M., Fuhriman, A., & Johnson, J. E. (2001). Cohesion in group psychotherapy. *Psychotherapy: Theory, Research, Practice, Training, 38*(4), 373–379.

Burns, D. D., & Spangler, D. L. (2000). Does psychotherapy homework lead to improvements in depression in cognitive-behavioral therapy or does improvement lead to increased homework compliance? *Journal of Consulting and Clinical Psychology, 68*(1), 46–56.

Cahalan, D., & Room, R. (1974). *Problem drinking among American men*. New Brunswick, NJ: Rutgers Center of Alcohol Studies.

Center for Substance Abuse Treatment. (1999). *Enhancing motivation for change in substance abuse treatment: Treatment improvement protocol (TIP) Series 35* (DHHS Publication No. SMA 99-3354). Rockville, MD: Substance Abuse and Mental Health Services Administration.

Center for Substance Abuse Treatment. (2005). *Substance abuse treatment: Group therapy. Treatment improvement protocol (TIP) Series 41* (DHHS Publication No. SMA 05-3991). Rockville, MD: Substance Abuse and Mental Health Services Administration.

Clifford, P. R., Maisto, S. A., & Davis, C. M. (2007). Alcohol treatment research assessment exposure subject reactivity effects: Part I. Alcohol use and related consequences. *Journal of Studies on Alcohol and Drugs, 68*(4), 519–528.

Connors, G. J., Carroll, K. M., DiClemente, C. C., Longabaugh, R., & Donovan, D. M. (1997). The therapeutic alliance and its relationship to alcoholism treatment participation and outcome. *Journal of Consulting and Clinical Psychology, 65*(4), 588–598.

Coviello, D. M., Alterman, A. I., Rutherford, M. J., Cacciola, J. S., McKay, J. R., & Zanis, D. A. (2001). The effectiveness of two intensities of psychosocial treatment for cocaine dependence. *Drug and Alcohol Dependence, 61*(2), 145–154.

Cummings, N. A., O'Donohue, W. T., & Ferguson, K. E. (2002). *The impact of medical cost offset on practice and research: Making it work for you.* Reno, NV: Context Press.

Cunningham, J. A., Sobell, M. B., Sobell, L. C., Gavin, D. R., & Annis, H. M. (1995). Heavy drinking and negative affective situations in a general population and a treatment sample: Alternative explanations. *Psychology of Addictive Behaviors, 9*(2), 123–127.

D'Amico, E. J., Feldstein Ewing, S. W., Engle, B., Hunter, S., Osilla, K. C., & Bryan, A. (2011). Group alcohol and drug treatment. In S. Naar-King & M. Suarez, *Motivational interviewing with adolescents and young adults* (pp. 151–157). New York: Guilford Press.

D'Amico, E. J., Osilla, K. C., & Hunter, S. B. (in press). Developing a group motivational interviewing intervention for adolescents at-risk for developing an alcohol or drug use disorder. *Alcoholism Treatment Quarterly.*

D'Onofrio, G., Bernstein, E., & Rollnick, S. (1996). Motivating patients for change: A brief strategy for negotiation. In E. Bernstein & J. Bernstein (Eds.), *Case studies in emergency room medicine and the health of the public* (pp. 295–303). Boston: Jones & Bartlett.

D'Zurilla, T. J., & Goldfried, M. R. (1971). Problem solving and behavior modification. *Journal of Abnormal Psychology, 78*, 107–126.

Davison, G. C. (2000). Stepped care: Doing more with less? *Journal of Consulting and Clinical Psychology, 68*(4), 580–585.

Dies, R. R. (1980). Group psychotherapy, training and supervision. In A. K. Hess (Ed.), *Psychotherapeutic supervision* (pp. 337–362). New York: Wiley.

Dies, R. R. (1992). The future of group therapy. *Psychotherapy, 29*, 58–64.

Dies, R. R. (1993). Research on group psychotherapy: Overview and clinical applications. In A. Alonso & H. I. Swiller (Eds.), *Group therapy in clinical practice* (pp. 473–518). Washington, D.C.: American Psychiatric Association Press.

Dies, R. R. (1994). The therapist's role in group treatments. In H. S. Bernard & K. R. MacKenzie (Eds.), *Basics of group psychotherapy* (pp. 60–99). New York: Guilford Press.

Duckert, F., Johnsen, J., & Amundsen, A. (1992). What happens to drinking after therapeutic intervention? *British Journal of Addiction, 87*(10), 1457–1467.

Dufour, M. C. (1999). What is moderate drinking? Defining "drinks" and drinking levels. *Alcohol Research and Health, 23*(1), 5–14.

Dunn, C., Deroo, L., & Rivara, F. P. (2001). The use of brief interventions adapted from motivational interviewing across behavioral domains: A systematic review. *Addiction, 96*(12), 1725–1742.

Edwards, G., Orford, J., Egert, S., Guthrie, S., Hawker, A., Hensman, C., et al. (1977). Alcoholism: A controlled trial of "treatment" and "advice." *Journal of Studies on Alcohol, 38*, 1004–1031.

Epstein, E. E., Drapkin, M. L., Yusko, D. A., Cook, S. M., McCrady, B. S., & Jensen, N. K. (2005). Is alcohol assessment therapeutic?: Pretreatment change in drinking among alcohol-dependent women. *Journal of Studies on Alcohol, 66*(3), 369–378.

Erickson, C. K. (2007). Let's not be afraid of harm reduction. *Addiction Professional, 5*(1), 10.

Feldman, D. J., Pattison, E. M., Sobell, L. C., Graham, T., & Sobell, M. B. (1975). Outpatient alcohol detoxification: Initial findings on 564 subjects. *American Journal of Psychiatry, 132*, 407–412.

Fleming, M. F., Barry, K. L., Manwell, L. B., Johnson, K., & London, R. (1997). Brief physician advice for problem alcohol drinkers: A randomized controlled trial in community-based primary care practices. *Journal of the American Medical Association, 227*, 1039–1045.

Forsyth, D. R. (2006). *Group dynamics* (4th ed.). Pacific Grove, CA: Brooks/Cole.

Foy, D. W., Nunn, L. B., & Rychtarik, R. G. (1984). Broad-spectrum behavioral treatment for chronic alcoholics: Effects of training controlled drinking skills. *Journal of Consulting and Clinical Psychology, 52*, 218–230.

French, M. T. (2000). Economic evaluation of alcohol treatment services. *Evaluation and Program Planning, 23*(1), 27–39.

Fuhriman, A., & Burlingame, G. M. (2001). Group psychotherapy training and effectiveness. *International Journal of Group Psychotherapy, 51*(3), 399–416.

Garland, A., & Scott, J. (2002). Using homework in therapy for depression. *Journal of Clinical Psychology, 58*(5), 489–498.

Gavin, D. R., Ross, H. E., & Skinner, H. A. (1989). Diagnostic validity of the Drug Abuse Screening Test in the assessment of the DSM-III drug disorders. *British Journal of Addiction, 84,* 301–307.

Gil, A. G., Wagner, E. F., & Tubman, J. G. (2004). Culturally sensitive substance abuse intervention for Hispanic and African American adolescents: Empirical examples from the Alcohol Treatment Targeting Adolescents in Need (ATTAIN) Project. *Addiction, 99,* 140–150.

Graham, K., Annis, H. M., Brett, P. J., & Venesoen, P. (1996). A controlled field trial of group versus individual cognitive-behavioural training for relapse prevention. *Addiction, 91*(8), 1127–1139.

Guimon, J. (2004). Evidence-based research studies on the results of group therapy: A critical review. *European Journal of Psychiatry, 18,* 49–60.

Harper, R., & Hardy, S. (2000). An evaluation of motivational interviewing as a method of intervention with clients in a probation setting. *British Journal of Social Work, 30*(3), 393–400.

Heather, N. (1989). Psychology and brief interventions. *British Journal of Addiction, 84,* 357–370.

Heather, N. (1999). Some common methodological criticisms of Project MATCH: Are they justified? *Addiction, 94*(1), 36–39.

Heather, N. (2005). Motivational interviewing: Is it all our clients need? *Addiction Research and Theory, 13*(1), 1–18.

Heather, N., & Robertson, I. (1981). *Controlled drinking.* London: Methuen.

Heather, N., Smailes, D., & Cassidy, P. (2008). Development of a readiness ruler for use with alcohol brief interventions. *Drug and Alcohol Dependence, 98*(3), 235–240.

Heimberg, R. G., & Becker, R. E. (2002). *Cognitive-behavioral group therapy for social phobia: Basic mechanisms and clinical strategies.* New York: Guilford Press.

Hofmann, S. G., & Suvak, M. (2006). Treatment attrition during group therapy for social phobia. *Journal of Anxiety Disorders, 20*(7), 961–972.

Holder, H., Longabaugh, R., Miller, W. R., & Rubonis, A. V. (1991). The cost effectiveness of treatment for alcoholism: A first approximation. *Journal of Studies on Alcohol, 52,* 517–540.

Hore, B. (1995). You can't just leave the goal choice to the patient. *Addiction, 90*(9), 1172–1173.

Horvath, A. O., & Luborsky, L. (1993). The role of the therapeutic alliance in psychotherapy. *Journal of Consulting and Clinical Psychology, 61*(4), 561–573.

Humphreys, K., Wing, S., McCarty, D., Chappel, J., Gallant, L., Haberle, B., et al. (2004). Self-help organizations for alcohol and drug problems: Toward evidence-based practice and policy. *Journal of Substance Abuse Treatment, 26*(3), 151–158.

Hunt, W. A., Barnett, L. W., & Branch, L. G. (1971). Relapse rates in addiction programs. *Journal of Clinical Psychology, 27,* 455–456.

Ingersoll, K. S., Wagner, C. C., & Gharib, S. (2002). *Motivational groups for community substance abuse programs.* Richmond, VA: Mid-Atlantic Addictions Technology Transfer Center.

Institute of Medicine. (1990). *Broadening the base of treatment for alcohol problems.* Washington, DC: National Academy Press.

International Center for Alcohol Policies. (1998, September). *International drinking guideline* (ICAP Report 14). Washington, DC: Author.

Janis, I. L., & Mann, L. (1977). *Decision-making: A psychological analysis of conflict, choice, and commitment.* New York: Free Press.

Kadden, R. M., Cooney, N. L., Getter, H., & Litt, M. D. (1989). Matching alcoholics to coping skills or interactional therapies: Posttreatment results. *Journal of Consulting and Clinical Psychology, 57,* 698–704.

Kahan, M. (1996). Identifying and managing problem drinkers. *Canadian Family Physician, 42,* 661–671.

Kalant, H. (1987). Nathan B. Eddy memorial award lecture: Tolerance and its significance for drug and alcohol dependence. *NIDA Research Monograph, 76,* 9–19.

Kaminer, Y. (2005). Challenges and opportunities of group therapy for adolescent substance abuse: A critical review. *Addictive Behaviors, 30*(9), 1765–1774.

Kanas, N., Stewart, P., Deri, J., Ketter, T., & Haney, K. (1989). Group process in short-term outpatient therapy groups for schizophrenics. *Group, 13,* 67–73.

Kazantzis, N. (2000). Power to detect homework effects in psychotherapy outcome research. *Clinical Psychology Review, 68*(1), 166–170.

Kazantzis, N., Deane, F. P., & Ronan, K. R. (2000). Homework assignments in cognitive and behavioral therapy: A meta-analysis. *Clinical Psychology: Science and Practice, 7*(2), 189–202.

Kazantzis, N., Deane, F. P., Ronan, K. R., & L'Abate, L. (2005). *Using homework assignments in cognitive-behavioral therapy.* New York: Routledge.

Kazantzis, N., & Shinkfield, G. (2007). Conceptualizing patient barriers to nonadherence with homework assignments. *Cognitive and Behavioral Practice, 14*(3), 317–324.

Kazdin, A. E. (2007). Mediators and mechanisms of change in psychotherapy research. *Annual Review of Clinical Psychology, 3*(1), 1–27.

Klingemann, H. K., & Sobell, L. C. (2007). *Promoting self-change from addictive behaviors: Practical implications for policy, prevention, and treatment.* New York: Springer.

Knight, K. M., McGowan, L., Dickens, C., & Bundy, C. (2006). A systematic review of motivational interviewing in physical health care settings. *British Journal of Health Psychology 11,* 319–332.

Lieber, C. S., Weiss, D. G., Groszmann, R., Paronetto, F., & Schenker, S. (2003). I. Veterans Affairs cooperative study of polyenylphosphatidylcholine in alcoholic liver disease: Effects on drinking behavior by nurse/physician teams. *Alcoholism: Clinical and Experimental Research, 27*(11), 1757–1764.

Linehan, M. M., Schmidt, H., Dimeff, L. A., Craft, J. C., Kanter, J., & Comtois, K. A. (1999). Dialectical behavior therapy for patients with borderline personality disorder and drug dependence. *American Journal on Addictions, 8*(4), 279–292.

Longabaugh, R., McCrady, B., Fink, E., Stout, R., McAuley, T., Doyle, C., et al. (1983). Cost-effectiveness of alcoholism treatment in partial vs. inpatient settings: Six-month outcomes. *Journal of Studies on Alcohol, 44,* 1049–1071.

MacKenzie, K. R. (1983). The clinical application of a group climate measure. In R. R. Dies & K. R. MacKenzie (Eds.), *Advances in group psychotherapy: Integrating research and practice* (pp. 159–170). New York: International Universities Press.

MacKenzie, K. R. (1994). The developing structure of the therapy group system. In H. S. Bernard & K. R. MacKenzie (Eds.), *Basics of group psychotherapy* (pp. 35–59). New York: Guilford Press.

MacKenzie, K. R. (1996). Time-limited group psychotherapy. *International Journal of Group Psychotherapy, 46*(1), 41–60.

MacKenzie, K. R. (1997). Advances in group psychotherapy. *Current Opinion in Psychiatry, 10*(3), 239–242.

Maisto, S. A., Henry, R. R., Sobell, M. B., & Sobell, L. C. (1978). Implications of acquired changes in tolerance for the treatment of alcohol problems. *Addictive Behaviors, 3*(1), 51–55.

Mann, L. (1972). Use of a "balance sheet" procedure to improve the quality of personal decision making: A field experiment with college applicants. *Journal of Vocational Behavior, 2,* 291–300.

Marijuana Treatment Project Research Group. (2004). Brief treatments for cannabis dependence: Findings from a randomized multisite trial. *Journal of Consulting and Clinical Psychology, 72*(3), 455–466.

Markland, D., Ryan, R. M., Tobin, V. J., & Rollnick, S. (2005). Motivational interviewing and self-determination theory. *Journal of Social and Clinical Psychology, 24*(6), 811–831.

Markus, H. E., & King, D. A. (2003). A survey of group psychotherapy training during predoctoral psychology internship. *Professional Psychology—Research and Practice, 34*(2), 203–209.

Marlatt, G. A., & Donovan, D. M. (Eds.). (2005). *Relapse prevention: Maintenance strategies in the treatment of addictive behaviors* (2nd ed.). New York: Guilford Press.

Marlatt, G. A., & Gordon, J. R. (Eds.). (1985). *Relapse prevention: Maintenance strategies in the treatment of addictive behaviors.* New York: Guilford Press.

Marlatt, G. A., Miller, W. R., Duckert, F., Goetestam, G., Heather, N., Peele, S., et al. (1985). Abstinence and controlled drinking: Alternative treatment goals for alcoholism and problem drinking? *Bulletin of the Society of Psychologists in Addictive Behaviors, 4*, 123–150.

Marques, A. C., & Formigoni, M. L. (2001). Comparison of individual and group cognitive-behavioral therapy for alcohol and/or drug-dependent patients. *Addiction, 96*(6), 835–846.

Martin, G. W., Herie, M. A., Turner, B. J., & Cunningham, J. A. (1998). A social marketing model for disseminating research-based treatments to addictions treatment providers. *Addiction, 93*(11), 1703–1715.

Martin, G. W., & Wilkinson, D. A. (1989). Methodological issues in the evaluation of treatment of drug dependence. *Advances in Behavioural Research and Therapy, 11*, 133–150.

Martino, S., Carroll, K. M., O'Malley, S. S., & Rounsaville, B. J. (2000). Motivational interviewing with psychiatrically ill substance abusing patients. *American Journal on Addictions, 9*(1), 88–91.

McKay, J. R., Alterman, A. I., Cacciola, J. S., Rutherford, M. J., O'Brien, C. P., & Koppenhaver, J. (1997). Group counseling versus individualized relapse prevention aftercare following intensive outpatient treatment for cocaine dependence: Initial results. *Journal of Consulting and Clinical Psychology, 65*(5), 778–788.

Meier, P. S., Barrowclough, C., & Donmall, M. C. (2005). The role of the therapeutic alliance in the treatment of substance misuse: A critical review of the literature. *Addiction, 100*(3), 304–316.

Miller, W. R. (1983). Motivational interviewing with problem drinkers. *Behavioural Psychotherapy, 11*, 147–172.

Miller, W. R. (1985). Motivation for treatment: A review with special emphasis on alcoholism. *Psychological Bulletin, 98*, 84–107.

Miller, W. R. (1986–1987). Motivation and treatment goals. *Drugs and Society, 1*, 133–151.

Miller, W. R. (2005). Motivational interviewing and the incredible shrinking treatment effect. *Addiction, 100*(4), 421.

Miller, W. R., & Brown, S. A. (1997). Why psychologists should treat alcohol and drug problems. *American Psychologist, 52*(12), 1269–1279.

Miller, W. R., & Rollnick, S. (1991). *Motivational interviewing: Preparing people to change addictive behavior.* New York: Guilford Press.

Miller, W. R., & Rollnick, S. (2002). *Motivational interviewing: Preparing people for change* (2nd ed.). New York: Guilford Press.

Miller, W. R., & Taylor, C. A. (1980). Relative effectiveness of bibliotherapy, individual and group self-control training in the treatment of problem drinkers. *Addictive Behaviors, 5*, 13–24.

Miller, W. R., & Wilbourne, P. L. (2002). Mesa Grande: A methodological analysis of clinical trials of treatments for alcohol use disorders. *Addiction, 97*(3), 265–277.

Mojtabai, R., & Zivin, J. G. (2003). Effectiveness and cost-effectiveness of four treatment modalities for substance disorders: A propensity score analysis. *Health Services Research, 38*(1), 233–259.

Monti, P. M., Abrams, D. B., Kadden, R. M., & Cooney, N. L. (1989). *Treating alcohol dependence: A coping skills training guide.* New York: Guilford Press.

Moran, A. P. (2004). *Sport and exercise psychology: A critical introduction.* New York: Routledge.

Morrison, M. (2001). Group cognitive therapy: Treatment of choice or sub-optimal option? *Behavioural and Cognitive Psychotherapy, 29*(3), 311.

Moyer, A., Finney, J. W., Swearingen, C. E., & Vergun, P. (2002). Brief interventions for alcohol problems: A meta-analytic review of controlled investigations in treatment-seeking and non-treatment-seeking populations. *Addiction, 97*(3), 279–292.

Moyers, T. B., Martin, T., Houck, J. M., Christopher, P. J., & Tonigan, J. S. (2009). From in-session behaviors to drinking outcomes: A causal chain for motivational interviewing. *Journal of Consulting and Clinical Psychology, 77*(6), 1113–1124.

Moyers, T. B., Miller, W. R., & Hendrickson, S. M. L. (2005). How does motivational interviewing work?: Therapist interpersonal skill predicts client involvement within motivational interviewing sessions. *Journal of Consulting and Clinical Psychology, 73*(4), 590–598.

Moyers, T. B., & Rollnick, S. (2002). A motivational interviewing perspective on resistance in psychotherapy. *Journal of Clinical Psychology, 58*(2), 185–193.

National Institute on Alcohol Abuse and Alcoholism. (1996). *How to cut down on your drinking*. Washington, DC: U.S. Government Printing Office.

National Institute on Alcohol Abuse and Alcoholism. (2007). *Helping patients who drink too much: A clinician's guide* (Updated 2005 ed.). Washington, DC: U.S. Government Printing Office.

Norcross, J. C., Hedges, M., & Prochaska, J. O. (2002). The face of 2010: A Delphi poll on the future of psychotherapy. *Professional Psychology: Research and Practice, 33*(3), 316–322.

Oei, T. P., & Jackson, P. (1980). Long-term effects of group and individual social skills training with alcoholics. *Addictive Behaviors, 5*, 129–136.

Orszag, P. (2008, January 31). *Congressional Budget Office Testimony: Growth in Health Care Costs*. Paper presented at the Committee on the Budget, United States Senate, Washington, DC.

Panas, L., Caspi, Y., Fournier, E., & McCarty, D. (2003). Performance measures for outpatient substance abuse services: Group versus individual counseling. *Journal of Substance Abuse Treatment, 25*(4), 271–278.

Perloff, R. M. (2008). *The dynamics of persuasion: Communication and attitudes in the 21st century* (3rd ed.). New York: Erlbaum.

Piper, W. E. (Ed.). (1993). *Group psychotherapy research*. Baltimore: Williams & Wilkins.

Piper, W. E., & Joyce, A. S. (1996). A consideration of factors influencing the utilization of time-limited, short-term group therapy. *International Journal of Group Psychotherapy, 46*, 311–328.

Prochaska, J. O., & DiClemente, C. C. (1982). Transtheoretical therapy: Toward a more integrative model of change. *Psychotherapy: Theory, Research and Practice 19*(3), 276–288.

Prochaska, J. O., & DiClemente, C. C. (1984). *The transtheoretical approach: Crossing traditional boundaries of therapy*. Homewood, IL: Dow Jones-Irwin.

Project MATCH. (1993). Project MATCH (Matching Alcoholism Treatment to Client Heterogeneity): Rationale and methods for a multisite clinical trial matching patients to alcoholism treatment. *Alcoholism: Clinical and Experimental Research, 17*(6), 1130–1145.

Project MATCH Research Group. (1997). Matching alcoholism treatments to client heterogeneity: Project MATCH posttreatment drinking outcomes. *Journal of Studies on Alcohol, 58*(1), 7–29.

Project MATCH Research Group. (1998). Matching alcoholism treatments to client heterogeneity: Project MATCH three-year drinking outcomes. *Alcoholism: Clinical and Experimental Research, 22*, 1300–1311.

Reinert, D. F., & Allen, J. P. (2007). The Alcohol Use Disorders Identification Test: An update of research findings. *Alcoholism, Clinical and Experimental Research, 31*(2), 185–199.

Resnicow, K., Dilorio, C., Soet, J. E., Borrelli, B., Hecht, J., & Ernst, D. (2002). Motivational interviewing in health promotion: It sounds like something is changing. *Health Psychology, 21*(5), 444–451.

Rogers, E. M. (1995). *Diffusion of innovations* (4th ed.). New York: Free Press.

Rollnick, S., & Allison, J. (2001). Motivational interviewing. In N. Heather, T. J. Peters, & T. Stockwell (Eds.), *International handbook of alcohol dependence and problems* (pp. 593–603). New York: Wiley.

Rollnick, S., & Miller, W. R. (1995). What is motivational interviewing? *Behavioural and Cognitive Psychotherapy, 23*, 325–334.

Rollnick, S., Miller, W. R., & Butler, C. C. (2008). *Motivational interviewing in health care: Helping patients change behavior*. New York: Guilford Press.

Rose, S. D. (1990). *Working with adults in groups: Integrating cognitive-behavioral and small group strategies*. San Francisco: Josey-Bass.

Rosenberg, S. A., & Zimet, C. N. (1995). Brief group treatment and managed mental health care. *International Journal of Group Psychotherapy, 45*, 367–379.

Sanchez-Craig, M. (1980). Random assignment to abstinence or controlled drinking in a cognitive-behavioral program: Short-term effects on drinking behavior. *Addictive Behaviors, 5*, 35–39.

Sanchez-Craig, M., Annis, H. M., Bornet, A. R., & MacDonald, K. R. (1984). Random assignment to abstinence and controlled drinking: Evaluation of a cognitive-behavioral program for problem drinkers. *Journal of Consulting and Clinical Psychology, 52*, 390–403.

Sanchez-Craig, M., Leigh, G., Spivak, K., & Lei, H. (1989). Superior outcome of females over males after brief treatment for the reduction of heavy drinking. *British Journal of Addiction, 84*, 395–404.

Sanchez-Craig, M., Spivak, K., & Davila, R. (1991). Superior outcome of females over males after brief treatment for the reduction of heavy drinking: Replication and report of therapist effects. *British Journal of Addiction, 86,* 867–876.

Santa Ana, E. J., Wulfert, E., & Nietert, P. J. (2007). Efficacy of group motivational interviewing (GMI) for psychiatric inpatients with chemical dependence. *Journal of Consulting and Clinical Psychology, 75*(5), 816–822.

Satterfield, J. M. (1994). Integrating group dynamics and cognitive-behavioral groups: A hybrid model. *Clinical Psychology: Science and Practice, 1*(2), 185–196.

Saunders, B., & Wilkinson, C. (1990). Motivation and addiction behaviour: A psychological perspective. *Drug and Alcohol Review, 9,* 133–142.

Scheidlinger, S. (1994). An overview of nine decades of group psychotherapy. *Hospital and Community Psychiatry, 45,* 217–225.

Schmitz, J. M., Oswald, L. M., Jacks, S. D., Rustin, T., Rhoades, H. M., & Grabowski, J. (1997). Relapse prevention treatment for cocaine dependence: Group vs. individual format. *Addictive Behaviors, 22*(3), 405–418.

Schoenholtz-Read, J. (1994). Selection of group intervention. In H. S. Bernard & K. R. MacKenzie (Eds.), *Basics of group psychotherapy* (pp. 157–188). New York: Guilford Press.

Schuckit, M. A., Smith, T. L., Danko, G. P., Bucholz, K. K., & Reich, T. (2001). Five-year clinical course associated with DSM-IV alcohol abuse or dependence in a large group of men and women. *American Journal of Psychiatry, 158*(7), 1084–1090.

Skinner, H. A. (1982). The Drug Abuse Screening Test. *Addictive Behaviors, 7,* 363–371.

Sklar, S. M., Annis, H. M., & Turner, N. E. (1997). Development and validation of the Drug-Taking Confidence Questionnaire: A measure of coping self-efficacy. *Addictive Behaviors, 22*(5), 655–670.

Sobell, L. C. (1996). Bridging the gap between scientists and practitioners: The challenge before us. *Behavior Therapy, 27*(3), 297–320.

Sobell, L. C., Kwan, E., & Sobell, M. B. (1995). Reliability of a Drug History Questionnaire (DHQ). *Addictive Behaviors, 20*(2), 233–241.

Sobell, L. C., & Sobell, M. B. (1973). A self-feedback technique to monitor drinking behavior in alcoholics. *Behaviour Research and Therapy, 11,* 237–238.

Sobell, L. C., & Sobell, M. B. (1995). Motivational strategies for promoting self-change: Dealing with alcohol and drug problems [Videotape]. Toronto, Ontario, Canada: Addiction Research Foundation.

Sobell, L. C., & Sobell, M. B. (2003). Alcohol consumption measures. In J. P. Allen & V. Wilson (Eds.), *Assessing alcohol problems* (2nd ed., pp. 75–99). Rockville, MD: National Institute on Alcohol Abuse and Alcoholism.

Sobell, L. C., Sobell, M. B., & Agrawal, S. (2009). Randomized controlled trial of a cognitive-behavioral motivational intervention in a group versus individual format for substance use disorders. *Psychology of Addictive Behaviors, 23*(4), 672–683.

Sobell, L. C., Sobell, M. B., Leo, G. I., Agrawal, S., Johnon-Young, L., & Cunningham, J. A. (2002). Promoting self-change with alcohol abusers: A community-level mail intervention based on natural recovery studies. *Alcoholism: Clinical and Expermental Research, 26,* 936–948.

Sobell, L. C., Wagner, E., Sobell, M. B., Agrawal, S., & Ellingstad, T. P. (2006). Guided self-change: a brief motivational intervention for cannabis users. In R. Roffman & R. Stephen (Eds.), *Cannabis dependence: Its nature, consequences, and treatment* (pp. 204–224). Cambridge, UK: Cambridge University Press.

Sobell, M. B., & Sobell, L. C. (1973). Individualized behavior therapy for alcoholics. *Behavior Therapy, 4,* 49–72.

Sobell, M. B., & Sobell, L. C. (1986–1987). Conceptual issues regarding goals in the treatment of alcohol problems. *Drugs and Society, 1,* 1–37.

Sobell, M. B., & Sobell, L. C. (1993a). *Problem drinkers: A guided self-change treatment.* New York: Guilford Press.

Sobell, M. B., & Sobell, L. C. (1993b). Treatment for problem drinkers: A public health priority. In J. S. Baer, G. A. Marlatt, & R. J. McMahon (Eds.), *Addictive behaviors across the lifespan: Prevention, treatment, and policy issues* (pp. 138–157). Beverly Hills, CA: Sage.

Sobell, M. B., & Sobell, L. C. (1995). Controlled drinking after 25 years: How important was the great debate? *Addiction, 90*, 1149–1153.

Sobell, M. B., & Sobell, L. C. (2000). Stepped care as a heuristic approach to the treatment of alcohol problems. *Journal of Consulting and Clinical Psychology, 68*(4), 573–579.

Sobell, M. B., & Sobell, L. C. (2005). Guided self-change treatment for substance abusers. *Journal of Cognitive Psychotherapy 19*, 199–210.

Sobell, M. B., Sobell, L. C., & Leo, G. I. (2000). Does enhanced social support improve outcomes got problem drinkers in guided self-change treatment? *Journal of Behavior Therapy and Experimental Psychiatry, 31*(1), 41–54.

Sobell, M. B., Sobell, L. C., & Gavin, D. R. (1995). Portraying alcohol treatment outcomes: Different yardsticks of success. *Behavior Therapy, 26*(4), 643–669.

Sobell, M. B., Sobell, L. C., & Sheahan, D. B. (1976). Functional analysis of drinking problems as an aid in developing individual treatment strategies. *Addictive Behaviors, 1*, 127–132.

Solomon, K. E., & Annis, H. M. (1990). Outcome and efficacy expectancy in the prediction of post-treatment drinking behaviour. *British Journal of Addiction, 85*, 659–665.

Spitz, H. I. (2001). Group psychotherapy of substance abuse in the era of managed mental health care. *International Journal of Group Psychotherapy, 51*(1), 21–41.

Stangier, U., Heidenreich, T., Peitz, M., Lauterbach, W., & Clark, D. M. (2003). Cognitive therapy for social phobia: Individual versus group treatment. *Behavior Research and Therapy, 41*(9), 991–1007.

Steenberger, B. T., & Budman, S. H. (1996). Group psychotherapy and managed behavioral health care: Current trends and future challenges. *International Journal of Group Psychotherapy, 46*, 297–309.

Stephens, R. S., Roffman, R. A., & Curtin, L. (2000). Comparison of extended versus brief treatments for marijuana use. *Journal of Consulting and Clinical Psychology, 68*(5), 898–908.

Stern, S. A., Meredith, L. S., Gholson, J., Gore, P., & D'Amico, E. J. (2007). Project CHAT: A brief motivational substance abuse intervention for teens in primary care. *Journal of Substance Abuse Treatment 32*(2), 153–165.

Stokes, J. P. (1983). Components of group cohesion: Intermember attraction, instrumental value, and risk taking. *Small Group Behavior, 14*, 163–173.

Substance Abuse and Mental Health Administration. (2003). *The ADSS cost study: Costs of substance abuse treatment in the speciality sector.* Rockville, MD: U.S. Department of Health and Human Services.

Suwaki, H., Kalant, H., Higuchi, S., Crabbe, J. C., Ohkuma, S., Katsura, M., et al. (2001). Recent research on alcohol tolerance and dependence. *Alcoholism, Clinical and Experimental Research, 25*(5 Suppl.), 189S–196S.

Swanson, A. J., Pantalon, M. V., & Cohen, K. R. (1999). Motivational interviewing and treatment adherence among psychiatric and dually diagnosed patients. *Journal of Nervous and Mental Disorders, 187*(10), 630–635.

Swift, R. M., & Miller, N. S. (1997). Integration of health care economics for addiction treatment in clinic care. *Journal of Psychoactive Drugs, 29*(3), 255–262.

Thorn, B. E. (2004). *Cognitive therapy for chronic pain: A step-by-step guide.* New York: Guilford Press.

Treadwell, T., Lavertue, N., Kumar, V., & Veeraraghavan, V. (2001). The Group Cohesion Scale—Revised: Reliability and validity. *International Journal of Action Methods: Psychodrama, Skill Training, and Role Playing, 54*(1), 3–11.

Tschuschke, V., Hess, H., & MacKenzie, K. R. (2002). GCQS Gruppenklima–Fragebogen [The Group Climate Questionnaire. GCQ-S]. In E. Brahler, J. Schymacher, & B. Straub (Eds.), *Diagnostische Verfahren in der Psychotherapie.* Göttingen, Germany: Hogrefe.

Tucker, M., & Oei, T. P. S. (2007). Is group more cost-effective than individual cognitive behaviour therapy? The evidence is not solid yet. *Behavior and Cognitive Psychotherapy, 35*(1), 77–91.

U.S. Department of Health and Human Services and U.S. Department of Agriculture. (2005). *Dietary guidelines for Americans, 2005* (6th ed.). Washington, DC: U.S. Government Printing Office.

Vakili, S., Sobell, L. C., Sobell, M. B., Simco, E. R., & Agrawal, S. (2008). Using the Timeline Followback to determine time windows representative of annual alcohol consumption with problem drinkers. *Addictive Behaviors, 33*(9), 1123–1130.

Vannicelli, M. (1992). *Removing the roadblocks: Group psychotherapy with substance abusers and family members.* New York: Guilford Press.

Walters, S., Vader, A., Harris, T. R., Field, C., & Jouriles, E. (2009). Dismantling motivational interviewing and feedback for college drinkers: A randomized clinical trial. *Journal of Consulting and Clinical Psychology, 77*(1), 64–73.

Walters, S. T., Bennett, M. E., & Miller, J. H. (2000). Reducing alcohol use in college students: A controlled trial of two brief interventions. *Journal of Drug Education, 30*(3), 361–372.

Walters, S. T., Ogle, R. O., & Martin, J. E. (2002). Perils and possibilities of group-based motivational interviewing. In W. R. Miller & S. Rollnick, *Motivational interviewing: Preparing people for change* (2nd ed., pp. 377–390). New York: Guilford Press.

Weiss, R. D., Jaffee, W. B., deMenil, V. P., & Cogley, C. B. (2004). Group therapy for substance use disorders: What do we know? *Harvard Review of Psychiatry, 12*(6), 339–350.

Wilkinson, D. A., Leigh, G. M., Cordingley, J., Martin, G. W., & Lei, H. (1987). Dimensions of multiple drug use and a typology of drug users. *British Journal of Addiction, 82,* 259–287.

Wilson, G. T. (1999). Rapid response to cognitive behavior therapy. *Clinical Psychology: Science and Practice, 6*(3), 289–292.

Witkiewitz, K., & Marlatt, G. A. (2004). Relapse prevention for alcohol and drug problems: That was Zen, this is Tao. *American Psychologist, 59*(4), 224–235.

Witkiewitz, K., & Marlatt, G. A. (2006). Overview of harm reduction treatments for alcohol problems. *International Journal of Drug Policy, 17*(4), 285–294.

Wright, J. H. (2004). *Cognitive-behavioral therapy.* Arlington, VA: American Psychiatric Publishing.

Yalom, I. (1985). *The theory and practice of group psychotherapy* (3rd ed.). New York: Basic Books.

Yalom, I., & Leszcz, M. (2005). *The theory and practice of group psychotherapy* (5th ed.). New York: Basic Books.

Index

Page numbers followed by *a* indicate appendix; *ch*, client handout; *f*, figure; *t*, table; and *th*, therapist handout

235